Health Care of the Older Adult

An Australian and New Zealand Nursing Perspective

Editor Dr. Peter Brown, Associate Professor of Nursing, School of Health Sciences, Charles Darwin University

16
EasyRead Large

RHYW

Copyright Page from the Original Book

Woodslane Press Pty Ltd
Unit 7/5 Vuko Place
Warriewood NSW 2102
Australia
Email: info@woodslane.com.au
Tel: (02) 9970 5111 Fax: (02) 9970 5002 www.woodslane.com.au

Health Care of the Older Adult

Print edition first published in 2010 by Woodslane Press
Ebook edition published by Woodslane Press in 2011

National Library of Australia Cataloguing-in-Publication entry

Editor: Brown, Dr. Peter, 1945-
Title: Health care of the Older Adult (electronic reference): an Australian and New Zealand nursing perspective / Dr. Peter Brown.
Edition: 1st ed.
ISBN: 9781921874024 (ebook)
Notes: Includes index.
Bibliography.
Subjects: Geriatric nursing—Australia.
Geriatric nursing—New Zealand.
Older people—Care—Australia.
Older people—Care—New Zealand.
Older people—Health and hygiene—Australia.
Older people—Health and hygiene—New Zealand.
Dewey Number: 610.73650994

Designed by Jenny Cowan

The table 'Person-centred care and personhood' on page 134, is from the article by Brendan McCormack entitled 'Person-centredness in Gerontological nursing: An overview of the literature' (Journal Clinical Nursing 2004, 13 [3A]), and is reproduced with the kind permission of Wiley-Blackwell

Set in 16 pt. Verdana

TABLE OF CONTENTS

About the Editor

The Editor, Dr. Peter Brown, has worked in various Universities in NSW over a 25 year span as a Lecturer, Senior Lecturer, and Assistant Head of School. Specialty content areas and interests include; mental health problems in old age, aged care, and mental health, having lectured in these specialties at undergraduate and post-graduate level. He has also lectured a multidisciplinary post-graduate course at the NSW Institute of Psychiatry. He has edited two textbooks on aged care and presented numerous conference papers, both nationally and internationally. Peter is a member of the Royal College of Nursing, Australia Health and Wellness in Ageing Faculty. He is currently Associate Professor in Clinical Practice, School of Health Sciences, Charles Darwin University. Peter's PhD focussed on older husbands' experience of providing care for wives with dementia at home.

Chapter 1

Ageing and care of the older adult

Dr. Peter Brown, RN, DNE, BHons, MA, PhD, MRCNA, ACMHN Associate Professor, School of Health Sciences, Charles Darwin University (CDU)

Objectives:

This chapter will enable the reader to:

1) develop an understanding of ageing and people's experience of ageing in our society;
2) identify 'myths' of ageing which are to be found in our society;
3) trace the development of interest in ageing from early times to the present;
4) examine the demographic profile of older adults in Australia and New Zealand (non-Indigenous and Indigenous);
5) develop an understanding of aged care provision in Australia and New Zealand; and
6) examine some of the important issues currently facing aged care and aged care nursing in Australia and New Zealand today.

Introduction

In this book you will examine the experiences of older adults as they age. But what is ageing? Ageing is defined in various ways and you might like to examine a dictionary definition (e.g. Macquarie, Oxford, Webster's) and a medical dictionary definition, and compare the definitions from these sources with one from a textbook on ageing or gerontological nursing, noting any contrasting ideas. In this chapter we will examine whether ageing is related to a particular chronological age or stage of life or more to the individual's level of functioning: What happens to body systems as we age? What is the level of interest in ageing in our society? Are we an ageing society? What health problems do older adults experience, and what is the nurse's role in relation to these? People aged 65 years and over are referred to by various descriptors; elderly, aged, older people and seniors to name a few. Currently, the most politically correct term is 'older adults'.

What is old age?

Life stages such as childhood and adulthood are socially constructed and are not fixed (Phillipson, 2001). These have been expanded and contracted in length and new ones have emerged in response to social changes and increasing knowledge (Degnen, 2006). We commonly identify *old age* as beginning at age 65 but this is not a recent invention. It reflects primarily the decision by various countries (e.g. European and the US) in the first half of the twentieth century to use this age to create their retirement or pension systems and determine eligibility for these benefits. Australia and New Zealand have followed this policy for many years as well (adult-life stages, http://family.jrank.org/pages/44/Adulthood-Life-Stages.html). Many authors feel that it is highly unsatisfactory and even inappropriate to fix mandatory retirement at 65 years of age, and more recently the Australian Government has encouraged older people to remain at work for longer (Australian Institute of Health and Welfare, 2007), introducing the provision of a bonus for each year past retirement age that the person stays in the workforce (the Australian Centre on Ageing).

In Chapter 4 biological changes associated with ageing are examined, but old age covers a greater range of years (65 to over 100) than any other age group and there are an increasing number of people living to over 100. It has been suggested, therefore, that we should divide old age up into at least four (or even more) groups: for example, young-old (65 to 74 years of age), middle-old (75 to 84), old-old (more than 85) and centenarians (over 100) (Meiner and Lueckenotte, 2006). Interestingly, there were 3,154 centenarians in Australia at the time of the 2006 Census and this number is expected to increase to 12,000 by the year 2020 (Richmond, 2008).

Where did our interest in ageing begin?

The first professions to develop education and practice orientations in relation to ageing were medicine, nursing, psychology and social work. Today, interest in ageing comes from a much broader representation of professions (Grabinski, 2007). Although somewhat dated now, Crandall (1991) has provided a very useful overview of the history of older adults in both preliterate and literate societies. According to Crandall, in preliterate societies older people were either well cared for or were treated poorly. Positive treatment was related to the special skills and information they possessed, and whether they performed a religious function. On the other hand, negative treatment was related to economic necessity (e.g. where the group was constantly on the move and didn't have time to provide for the sick, older members etc.), less societal complexity (e.g. lacking infrastructure to manage elderly, sick etc.) and political roles (e.g. their place in society was taken over by others, often younger members).

Look at the following propositions about older people and compare them with what you know about older adults in our society. *In what ways are the characteristics similar/different?*

- they are a minority group
- women significantly outnumber men and there is a high proportion of widows

- they fill age-specific roles (e.g. retirees, volunteers, carers)
- they leave the economic workforce and take on other roles
- a few continue in political, judicial, business and civic roles
- they are looked after by their adult children
- they seek methods to prolong life

Socio-demographics of old age

Although a minority group still, the number of older adults will continue to grow as a proportion of the total Australian and New Zealander populations. Similarly, when examining OECD countries (e.g. UK, Sweden etc.), we find that older adults comprise a significant and growing proportion of their populations. Indeed many of these countries have a higher proportion of older adults (Parliament of Australia, 2006) than Australia and New Zealand (AIHW, 2007). We will see a similar trend in Australia and New Zealand over time.

In Australia and New Zealand there are more widows than widowers (AIHW, 2007). However, unlike earlier societies it is probably not true that men in our society leave the economic workforce and enter advisory or supervisory roles in our society, although some will do this. In earlier times older adults were more directly looked after by adult children but in our own society it is still not common to have more than one or two generations living in the same household.

Adult children in our society, however, provide a lot of indirect support by telephoning on a regular basis, visiting and providing hospitality for older mothers and fathers.

Many writers have argued that until more recent years there has been little interest in older people and ageing. *Consider what this was related to.*

Perhaps you identified one or more of the following explanations.

1) Low numbers due to shortened life expectancy
2) Old age was not seen as a separate stage of life (subsumed under adulthood)
3) Older people were not viewed as a group with specialised needs
4) Stigma associated with being old
5) Professionals' interest in older people was limited as:
   a) education focussed on the young;
   b) personality was seen as developing at a young age;
   c) within medicine/biology, older people were not seen as being sufficiently interesting as a dramatic 'cure' was not possible and highlighted failure of skills;
   d) it highlighted health professionals' own negative attitudes toward their own ageing and death;
   e) political scientists were interested only in their voting patterns, party affiliation and political attitudes;

f) anthropologists used them as informants about a particular society's history, beliefs and practices;

g) old age was even viewed itself as being 'a disease'

(Crandall, 1991; Phillipson, 2001; Grabinski, 2007).

Studies by Crandall (1991), Birren and Schaie (2001), Phillipson (2001) and Phillipson and Scarf (2004) have proposed that changes in interest in ageing and older adults were related to a number of factors, including:

- the increasing numbers of older people;
- the rise of the union movement and its involvement in the introduction of pensions and superannuation;
- increased interest in the phenomenon of 'stigma';
- changes in educational thinking (emphasis is now on lifelong learning and people moving in and out of the educational system during their life time as and when needed);
- development of the lifecycle approach to the study of physiological, psychological and sociological experiences of all individuals;
- interest in what they could continue to contribute to society;
- creation of lectureships, professorial chairs (e.g. http://www.rsllifecare.org.au) and research posts;
- development of nurse practitioners in aged care (Paterson, Xiao, Mitchell, Henderson, De Bellis and Kelton, 2007);

- gerontological health professionals confronting their own ageing (Ebersole, Hess, and Luggen, 2004).

Old age (or late adulthood)

Unfortunately, ageing is not something we can easily avoid. It begins at conception and ends in death. It is a process of growing older in which mental and physical decline occurs. It is a universal experience and species specific (we live, as the old saying goes, 'three score years and 10', but crocodiles may live for 100 years while some tortoises may live for hundreds of years). When we examine the available statistics we find that, in Australia, females live on average for 82 years and males 76 years (Australian Bureau of Statistics, 2003). Average life expectancy is predicted to increase to 88.1 years for females and 82.9 for males by 2027 (Booth and Tickle, 2003). This infers that there is a gender difference in how long men and women live. *Try to find out why.*

Hopefully in your research you will have identified that one of the factors conducive to ageing is related to biology. Santrock (2006, p.556) identifies that women's oestrogen production provides some protection against arteriosclerosis and their extra X chromosome may be associated with greater antibody production compared to men. Elsewhere, it has been suggested that women's hearts age more slowly than men's (Medical News, 2005). Santrock (2006, p.557), after reviewing other researchers, suggests that it is not only related to genetics but also to a greater ability to cope with stress, health, education, personality and lifestyle. *Do you think that women are able to 'handle' more stressors than men? Why? Why not?*

Santrock (2006, p.555) defines life expectancy as the number of years that will probably be lived by the average person who is born in a particular year. We are currently witnessing a greater number of people living into old age and into old-old age. *How do you account for this phenomenon? What is your life expectation?* (see gosset.wharton.upenn.edu/mortality/perl/CalcForm.html.)

You will probably have identified factors such as improvements in medicine, nutrition, exercise, occupation and lifestyle, including reduction in smoking behaviour.

The other term that Santrock (2006, p.555) defines is *lifespan.* By this he means the maximum number of years an individual can live. Interestingly, and as we have already seen, there are significantly more people living to 100 years or more and this number will only continue to increase. In an article in The Bulletin on 23/1/2006, National Affairs Editor Tony Wright stated that the average lifespan '...will double over the next seven to 10 years and keep doing so. In short, there will likely be 12,000 centenarians in Australia by 2020, and 50,000 by 2050'. The interesting thing about this trend is that it will occur when Australia's total population may be in decline. In the light of this phenomenon, consider the statement *'The older you are the sicker you get'.*

As we have seen, some gerontologists categorise older people in terms of chronological age (e.g. young-old, middle-old, old-old and centenarians). Others prefer to talk about ageing in terms of function, proposing that ageing affects us at every level, including biologically, socially, psychologically and cognitively. An interesting concept here is that each older person may be functioning at their stated age, or younger or even older. *Can you think of an example of this?* In addition, changes in function do not always proceed symmetrically, so that an older adult may be very good cognitively but may be experiencing various physical problems to a greater or lesser extent. *How do you account for this phenomenon?*

Ageing in Australia

There are about 2.3 million older adults aged 65 and over (or 13% of the population) in Australia and the proportion is growing. The population of Australia is clearly ageing as evidenced by Table 1 (AIHW, 2007 Demographic profile: Older Australians at a glance. h ttp://www.aihw.gov.au/publications/age/oag04/oag0 4-c01.pdf).

Table 1: Increases in the Australian older population over time

Year	Percentage of population
65 years of age and over	
1999	12.2%
2036	24%
80 years of age and over	

Year	Percentage of population
2006	3.6%
2036	7.9%
85 years of age and over	
2001	1.3%
2051	1.6%

(AIHW, 2007)

Clearly, the number of older people as a proportion of Australia's total population is increasing over time, but what has accounted for these observable increases? Possible answers include Australia's migration policy, decreased mortality rates (and high quality public and clinical health programs) and increased fertility rates (high birth rates). What we are seeing by and large is the effect of larger fertility rates in earlier generations so that greater numbers of people are moving through into old age during our lifetime. Currently, we know that fertility rates are much lower and therefore in the future, as smaller numbers of current children enter old age, there will be a stabilisation and/or decrease in the numbers of older people as a proportion of the total population (Parliament of Australia, 2003).

In Australia, there are 75 men for every 100 women aged 65 and over, and 40 men for every 100 women over the age of 85. Thirteen percent of people aged over 65 were born overseas. Of these, 80% were originally from a non-English speaking background (e.g. Italy, Greece, Germany or China). Aboriginal and Torres Strait Islanders have a lower life expectancy than the general population and represent only 4% of the total population (AIHW, 2007). *Why do you think this might be so?*

Diversity of the aged population

In earlier times, older adults were perceived by some as being more homogeneous (that is, they were seen as being similar to each other) than heterogeneous (that is, markedly different from each other), but with a greater understanding of the older population it is clear that they are as heterogeneous as any other age group in the population. We can note the following differences: women outnumber men (especially those 85 years of age and over); older adults' experiences in rural areas are very different from those of their counterparts in metropolitan areas; a significant number of older people come from different culturally and linguistically diverse backgrounds; Indigenous Australians aged over 65 comprise 3.3% of all Indigenous Australians (ABS, 2006). It is a sad indictment that only just over 15,000 Indigenous Australians are aged 65 and over (0.56% of all Australians aged 65 and over (AIHW, 2007)). Additionally, life expectancy at birth in 2001 for Indigenous Australians was on average of 17 years less than life expectancy for Australia as a whole. Indigenous Australians are therefore considered to be 'older adults' at 50 years of age (AIHW, 2007).

Older people from culturally and linguistically diverse (CALD) backgrounds comprised approximately one in four older Australians in 1996. By 2006, they comprised one in three (AIHW, 2007). This high number of older people from CALD backgrounds is related to Australia's post-war immigration policies, which encouraged higher levels of immigration, and more recent policies which encouraged greater numbers of older immigrants from overseas countries (e.g. UK, China, India, Philippines, Vietnam) (AIHW, 2007).

Just over half of those Australians 65 years and over have some form of disability, with significantly higher numbers coming from those 80 years of age and over (40% of females compared to 27% of males). Single older people are more reliant on government pensions than couples. Most older adults live independently and it is worth noting that only 6% live in nursing homes, hostels and retirement villages, with 3% in non-private dwellings (e.g. hospitals). Of those older adults who live in private dwellings, most (62%) live with spouses or partners while 28% live alone, and the proportion of women living alone increases with age (*Australia's older people. Demographic issues and population ageing.* http://www.aic.gov.au/publications/rpp/32/older.pdf).

Ageing in New Zealand

As of 18 July 2009, there were an estimated resident population of 4,319,239 and an estimated population growth of 43,700, including a net migration gain of 10,100. The Maori ethnic group was estimated to be 632,900. Those aged 65 years and over made up 12.5% of the New Zealand population (Statistics New Zealand, Demographic trends 2007 (a)) and are expected to rise to 24% (or 1.41 million) of the population in 2041 (Population Ageing in New Zealand, 2006). One in 8 people are aged 65 years and over (Statistics New Zealand, Census Snapshot 2007, b.). Males and females aged 90 years and over recorded the largest growth during the decade 1997 to 2007. Women continue to outnumber men in the older age groups (e.g. there were two thirds more women aged 80 years and over than there were men). The life expectancy at birth was 81.9 for women and 77.9 years for men. However, there are some regional differences in life expectancy with Auckland, Wellington, Tasman, Canterbury and Otago all experiencing above average life expectancies over the last decade, while other regions (e.g. Bay of Plenty, West Coast and Southland) recorded life expectancies below the national average. The latter has been attributed to the proportion of the populations who are Maori, extent of urbanisation and closeness to health services. Maori life expectancy is, therefore, significantly lower than the life expectancy of the total population (69 years for men and 73.2 for women) (Ministry of Health, 2002; Statistics New Zealand, Demographic trends 2007 (c)).

Number of overseas-born Australians and New Zealanders

In New Zealand in 2006, 23.1% of older adults had been born overseas and this is expected to rise to 26.3% of the older population by 2051. Of these, the majority are European in origin (Statistics New Zealand, 2004).

Implications of an ageing population

Older people must be enabled to make continuing contributions to our community. With a recent increase in workforce participation by older workers, older adults will continue to share their knowledge, skills and experiences with younger employees (Australian Institute of Health and Welfare, 2007). In addition, their continuing spending power will increase economic growth. However, older workers who have lost their jobs will find it difficult to find re-employment because of age discrimination (Encel and Studencki, 2004). Older adults will eventually become major users of aged care and health services and governments will need to ensure that services are of high quality and appropriate to their needs. Recruitment, retention and education of staff in aged care will require adequate responses from governments and the private sector. Policies must also encourage health promotion, education and social participation (AIHW, 2007).

Health of older adults in Australia and New Zealand

Unfortunately, as the populations of both Australia and New Zealand age, an increasing number of older adults will develop adverse health conditions, disability and decreased health status (Ministry of Health, 2002; ABS, 2004). Commonly reported health conditions in Australia are diseases of the eyes, musculoskeletal conditions and circulatory system, osteoarthritis, and respiratory conditions. Accidental falls increase with age (ABS, 2004). New Zealand figures indicate that incidences of ischaemic heart disease, stroke, respiratory diseases and lung cancer and other cancers increase with age (Ministry of Health, 2002). Health problems of older people are discussed in more detail in Chapters 6 and 7.

Aged care services in New Zealand

Residential aged care services in New Zealand include:

- Retirement villages – multi-storied complexes comprising residential units, medium dependency and possibly high-level rest home beds
- Rest homes – providing medium dependency beds and possibly high-level private hospital and dementia care beds

- Private hospitals – providing private hospital and dementia care beds
- Ancillary retirement complexes – serviced apartments and eco-villages (see, for example, http://www.converge.org.nz/evcnz/archive/index_sum01.html) (Lazonby, 2007)

In 2005, it was estimated that approximately 30,000 older adults lived in residential aged care facilities (Bland, 2005). Bland, a New Zealand researcher, highlights the challenges associated with becoming a nursing home resident while then trying to establish a new sense of 'home'. The challenge for nurses in aged care facilities is to develop an understanding of the unique story of each resident.

Community or domiciliary nursing services in New Zealand is provided through 21 District Health Boards and these offer contracts to providers of home-based services. Nurses may have a range of specialist roles. In addition, community health nurses may work for government services (Murray and Lewis, 2008).

Aged care services in Australia

Community care

Most older Australians prefer to stay in their own homes, so there are a number of programs available to help out with daily living activities that may have become harder to manage on their own. This is called 'community care'. The Home and Community Care program (HACC) and the Community Aged Care

Packages (CACP) are two such programs, with services specifically designed for older Australians who would qualify for at least low-level care in an aged care home. CACP provides a package of services whereas HACC may provide one or more services (Australian Government, 2009).

HACC services aim to meet basic needs to maintain older adults' independence at home and in the community, including community nursing, domestic assistance, personal care, meals on wheels, home modification and maintenance, transport and community-based respite care. The Extended Aged Care at Home (EACH) and Extended Aged Care at Home Dementia (EACH D) programs also provide services for high-level care needs at home. Eligibility for CACP, EACH and EACH D is assessed by Aged Care Assessment Teams (ACATs or Aged Care Assessment Service in Victoria) (Parliament of Australia, 2003).

Bruen (2005) argues that the demand for community care for older people will only continue to increase and will include expansion of support from family carers, externally-provided community care and age friendly housing. The challenge, of course, will be determining who will fund this and what proportion will be funded by government versus users of the services.

Aged care homes

If the older person cannot live at home because of illness or disability, there are publicly-funded places in aged care homes that may be accessed. This is called 'residential aged care'. There are two types of residential aged care in Australia – high-level and low-level care. High-level care provides nursing care when required, meals, laundry, cleaning and personal care, while low-level care gives assistance with meals, laundry and personal care only when required. To be eligible for either of these aged care places the older person needs to be assessed by an Aged Care Assessment Team (Australian Government Department of Health and Ageing).

Role of the nurse in aged care

Over recent years, radical changes have occurred in aged care. These changes have implications for the role of the nurse and for the ways in which nurses are educated. Changes include a significant increase in the number of older adults in the Australian and New Zealand populations. We can also note that old age is not a curable condition, and the traditional medical model of care is therefore not wholly appropriate for their care. In addition, we probably should be using terms like wellness (living life to the full) rather than 'experiencing health free of disease', 'sub-clinical conditions' or 'age-related changes and effects'. However, ageing should not be equated with disease. When nurses and others fully realise this, older adults will no longer be seen as 'objects of care' and the nurse's focus of attention will be on the older person's functional status rather than trying to 'cure' them – this only results in frustration and is based on a fundamental misunderstanding of what is really happening. It implies that aged care nursing will probably not involve high technology, be fast paced or action-oriented. It also means that it may not be as exciting as working in a high-dependency hospital facility (depending, of course, on how you define 'exciting'!). For many older adults, their health care needs will be chronic. For those doctors and nurses whose treatment orientation is to 'cure' patients, aged care may not appeal as there may be no cure as such or reaching one may take much longer. This does not mean, of course, that older people will not develop acute illnesses (see chapters 6 and 7) which may be curable quite quickly.

Older people may be nursed in an acute hospital setting, and some (although not as many as might be perceived) will live in low (approximately 12%) and high care facilities (approximately 8%) (Benevolent Society, 2007). Others will be nursed with various levels of support in the community, including community care and transition care (Department of Health and Ageing, 2008).

Nursing older people is a specialised area of nursing practice. One of the reasons for this is that symptom presentation related to disease processes in older people may not present with typical presentations. This means that geriatricians (medical doctors working with older people), psychogeriatricians (doctors who have training in medical and psychiatric problems occurring in old age), aged care (or gerontological) nurses (nurses who work with older people with medical problems) and psychogeriatric nurses (nurses who work with older people with psychiatric problems) have to be very good detectives. This type of care requires the development of a sufficient knowledge base which allows specialist nurses in aged care to use their clinical judgements effectively in the care of older adults.

Geriaction (a professional Australian organisation) has developed competency standards for advanced practice in gerontological nursing. The content of these standards was drawn from the findings of a longitudinal research study undertaken by the organisation which aimed to gain views on generic advanced nurse competencies from a wide range of expert aged care nurses in Australia. Findings resulted in the identification of 12 nursing standards, each including between seven and 12 elements that illustrated the specificity of gerontological nursing within each standard. These are identified in the publication *Competency Standards for the Advanced Gerontological Nurse.* Sydney: John Thrift Publishing, 2000. The 12 standards are as follows:

1) Uses multiple approaches to decision making
2) Manages the care of older persons
3) Engages in collaborative practice to achieve the positive outcomes for older persons
4) Provides support and development for colleagues and other members of the health care team

5) Manages the utilisation of staff and physical resources
6) Engages in ethically justifiable nursing practice
7) Advocates and protects the rights of older persons
8) Engages in practices to improve gerontological nursing practice
9) Develops therapeutic caring relationships
10) Fulfils the conduct requirement of the profession
11) Acts to enhance the professional development of self
12) Functions in accordance with legislation and common law affecting nursing practice

Reed, Inglis, Cook, Clarke and Clarke (2001) suggests that gerontological nurse specialists should possess a number of key attributes, including holistic knowledge and practice, familiarity with the patient, moral agency and skilled know how.

Consider these competencies/attributes in relation to any experiences you may have had in aged care. Which ones have you seen in practice? Which ones have you not seen? Are there other competencies that you think have been left out? If so, what are they?

An important focus of aged care nursing must also be to encourage the practice of health-related behaviours by older adults. It is not difficult to see that this emphasis will be an important approach for community aged care nurses. It is not as easy to accept that a health promotion role can also be practised in a high care aged care facility. *Provide several examples of what could be done for older adults in high care.*

Of course, health promotion and preventative health care will not halt the ageing process, but it may reduce the effects of existing problems and prevent further complications and dependency. Clearly, we can observe from our own experience that most older adults are healthy and living at home (Australian Bureau of Statistics, 2004). For those older adults experiencing chronic and disabling conditions, health promotion should be directed towards keeping them healthy in day-to-day functioning. For example, approaching retirement with a positive attitude, paying attention to nutritional and dietary needs, achieving a balance between exercise and rest and keeping mentally and physically active will assist the older adult to stay generally healthy, and those with chronic and disabling conditions as well as possible. So even where the older adult is experiencing a chronic illness it is possible to achieve and maintain optimal wellness. But what is 'wellness' in this context? Basically, it is adapting to whatever one is faced with (e.g. ill health) so as to achieve as much health as possible while at the same time being realistic about one's capabilities (Ebersole, Hess and Luggen, (2004; Meiner and Lueckenotte, 2006). *What do you think of this idea?*

Commitment to aged care nursing

So what does a commitment to the development of aged care nursing specialisation mean? Reviewing the literature, there are a number of indicators that highlight how well we are developing as a specialty. These indicators include: the number of gerontological nursing textbooks and journals focusing exclusively on gerontological nursing; articles on aged care in general nursing journals; published research articles on various aspects of aged care; national and international conferences focusing on aged care nursing education, research and practice; post-graduate nursing courses in aged care nursing offered by tertiary institutions; the appointment of Aged Care Professors and the development of Teaching Nursing Homes.

Attracting nurses to aged care

A key challenge for the aged care industry is how to attract nurses into aged care and how to retain them. Much of the research literature indicates that nursing students and nurses generally are not interested. Stevens and Crouch (1992) surveyed 610 beginning nursing students on their orientation day in 14 undergraduate (UG) nursing courses in New South Wales universities. Study findings indicated that aged care was of low interest to beginning students.

Perhaps one of the explanations for the above findings is that it highlights the phenomenon of 'ageism'. Basically, ageism is a prejudice concerned with ignorance, being deprived of power and stereotypes (Eliopoulos, 2004). Nurses and other health workers are sometimes ageist without really realising that it is happening to them. The problem here, of course, is that such an attitude may affect their attitudes towards older adults and even impact on the level of care provided, while limiting their expectations of older patients or clients. Hence many graduates from UG nursing courses enter their new graduate hospital-based programmes to facilitate this perceived need.

Elsewhere, Henderson, Xiao, Siegloff, Kelton and Paterson (2008) found that commencing undergraduate nursing students generally had positive attitudes towards older people but did not aspire to work with them. Where there were negative perceptions in evidence it was reported to be related to associating ageing with loss of physical and mental function.

This idea finds support in findings from Courtney, Tong and Walsh (2000), who were interested to examine acute care nurses' attitudes towards older patients in an Australian context. Findings indicated that negative attitudes towards older patients resulted in reduced independence, limited decision-making opportunities and little consideration of their age-related needs.

Elsewhere, Rognstad, Aasland and Granum (2004) studied first year nurse students' motivations and beliefs in relation to nursing work. Their findings highlighted that most preferred a nursing job where they could undertake further specialist study, experience human contact and assist others. Surprisingly, given this finding, students' preferences did not incorporate an interest in working with the chronically ill and older adults. The authors suggested that this finding was related to societal attitudes which associate personal success with health and fitness. Similarly, Herdman (2002) found that student nurses selected specialty areas they believed would enhance their clinical skills after graduation, as well as future prospects.

Swedish researchers Soderhamn, Lindencrona and Gustavsson (2001) attempted to identify factors that were associated with student nurses and registered nurses showing less favourable feelings towards older adults. Findings indicated that these were associated with limited experience caring for older people, being less than 25 years of age and being male. The authors noted that their findings were consistent with those reported elsewhere. Ideas provided by the researchers to address these findings included early clinical experiences in aged care in under-graduate nursing courses and positive role modelling by nursing academic staff members (especially males).

Perhaps not surprisingly, undergraduate nursing students have found clinical placements in aged care unsatisfactory and, for some, unsettling (Abbey, Abbey, Bridges, Elder, Lemcke, Liddle and Thornton, 2006). Consequently, few graduates choose to explore aged care as an employment option. Factors involved in lack of interest include unexamined assumptions of old age, lack of pre-clinical orientation and supervision and status, income and career pathway limitations (Abbey et al., 2006). Wallace, Brown, Cumming and Waugh (2007), Australian researchers, found that an arrangement like the Teaching Nursing Home (see http://teachingnursinghomes.com) could lead to more positive attitudes towards working in aged care, increase collaborative research activities and increase the number of staff undertaking post-graduate studies.

Nurses and older adults' health and wellness

The concept of health has been variously defined in the literature. Being healthy involves ongoing adjustment to stressors (both internal and external) by using personal and other resources to achieve a sense of wellbeing. When we consider the changes that occur with ageing, perhaps a good definition of health in this situation is the ability of older adults to function at their highest level of functioning despite these changes (see the concept of *wellness* described earlier in this chapter). According to Peel, Bartlett and McClure (2004) healthy ageing is the capacity to function well and adapt to environmental challenges in all domains, i.e., physical, mental and social. Elsewhere (http://www.seniors.gov.au.senior.gov.au), healthy ageing is defined by describing the ongoing activities and behaviours the older adult undertakes to reduce becoming ill and increase physical, emotional and mental health. It also includes the concept of reducing the impact of illness and disease through lifestyle changes so as to hasten recovery and prevent relapse. However, there is a real sense that health may be defined differently by individual older people, so that one older adult equates health with having intimate interpersonal relationships with others, whereas another older person might perceive health as being physically fit. The World Health Organisation's definition of health stresses that as age increases, diagnostic labels reduce in importance and the person's level of functioning and sense of wellbeing assumes more significance (Miller, 2009). Increasingly, older adults also associate health with their ability to function or perform certain tasks (e.g. exercising, eating, sleeping, socialising). Age alone, therefore, is not an adequate predictor of health status and one's definition of health changes with age. Stanley and Beare (2005), therefore, propose that health in ageing is a state of mind in older adults even where their bodies may be breaking down.

Spend a few minutes thinking about the following statement: *'It is too late for older adults to benefit from changing their lifelong unhealthy habits'.*

Health promotion

Health promotion is important to older adults as it can assist in modifying risk factors, slowing down the effects of the ageing process and enhancing the quality of the remaining years of life. An important nursing responsibility will be to encourage older adults to assume greater responsibility for their own wellness (Allied and Scientific Health Office, 2009). Health promotion and preventative health care will not halt the ageing process but may reduce the negative effects of existing problems and prevent further complications and therefore dependency. It aims to increase the level of wellbeing of the older adult, actualising their health potential while encouraging them to achieve and maintain a greater level of wellbeing (Meiner and Lueckenotte, 2006), physically, psychologically, emotionally, socially and spiritually. However, it is not being suggested that the older adult will be free from existing disease or disability.

Prevention

Health promotion and disease prevention includes concepts such as primary and secondary prevention. Primary prevention involves prevention of disease before it occurs. Secondary prevention includes detection of disease at an early stage in its development (Resnick, 2003).

Primary prevention includes dietary measures such as low-fat diets, regular exercise, smoking cessation, moderate use of alcohol, stress reduction, participating in computer workshops and belonging to the University of the Third Age (U3A) (see http://www3.griffith.edu.au/03/u3a/; Burban k, Padula and Nigg, 2000). Russell, Campbell and Hughes (2008) found that older internet users were able to enhance their connections with friends and family while engaging with wider social networks (see also Irizarry, West and Downing, 2001). Secondary prevention includes measures such as biennial mammography, clinical breast examinations, self-breast examinations, cervical smears, screening for skin lesions and faecal occult blood and prostate examination. According to Resnick (2003), screening in the elderly depends on: (1) whether the disease/condition will impact on the quality of life, (2) whether treatment is an acceptable option and (3) the implications of delaying treatment.

Acceptance of health promotional activities by older people may depend on a number of factors including: (1) socioeconomic factors, (2) beliefs and attitudes of both patients and providers, (3) encouragement by a health provider, (4) specific motivation based on efficacy beliefs and (5) access to resources (Resnick, 2003). Unfortunately for many of advancing age there is less willingness to participate in health promoting activities.

Role of the nurse in relation to retirement, nutrition and physical activity

The nurse has a key role in incorporating health promoting strategies into older patient care in both hospital and community settings. Imamura's (2002) study, located in a government-assisted apartment complex in the US, included 143 low-income elderly adults. Of these, a total of 55 elderly people participated in health promotion programmes entitled 'Amy's Chat Room'. Participants had a range of health problems. Topics discussed during three meetings included chronic diseases and their prevention, healthy eating, lifelong exercise and relaxation. Unfortunately, only a small number of elderly people living in the complex attended all three meetings. Of those who did attend, however, the majority requested future meetings on health-related topics. Australian researchers Bates, Donaldson, Lloyd, Castell, Krolik and Coleman (2009) have reported that on a weekly basis, community-based strength programs show promise in improving older adults' functional capacity, including their strength. In the UK, Cattan, White, Bond and Learmouth (2005) have proposed that educational and social activity groups can alleviate social isolation and loneliness among older adults. Findings of a study by Barnett, Smith, Lord, Williams and Baumand

(2003), which aimed to test whether community-based exercise reduced falls in at-risk older people, highlighted that older participants experienced less postural sway and coordinated stability.

Retirement

Retirement is a time for major readjustments in all aspects of the older person's life. It has been a common practice for men in Australia to retire at 65 and women at 60 years of age. Increasingly, many people in the workforce have experienced early retrenchment. An increasing number of people will enter into retirement unwillingly. Retirement, therefore, may be viewed negatively for people in this situation (Australian Government, 2006). Others may be pressured into retiring by their spouses. The time spent in retirement for many will be considerable. For many people retirement will be a happy period in their lives but for others it will be stressful experience. Factors associated with life satisfaction in retirement are good general and mental health (Australian Government, 2006). Not only has the person lost their job, but they may experience reductions in income, influence, social relationships, activity and professional skills. For many older adults, there will be a significant increase in unstructured time.

Over the years retirement has been more of a crisis for men as in previous generations men have been the 'breadwinners' while women stayed at home as wives and mothers. But, with more women entering and staying in the workforce they too will experience problems in greater numbers associated with retirement. It is not difficult to perceive how this new relationship might create difficulties for both wives and husbands.

Imagine if the retiree was obsessively tied to work. It is not difficult in this situation to see that such an individual will experience a strong sense of loss upon retiring. Equally the person with perfectionist tendencies who has difficulty accepting his own accomplishments may also experience retirement in a negative way. Income reduction will for many cause undue stress. From a health promotion perspective, planning for retirement is an important issue. Ideally, one should have paid off their mortgage, belong to a retirement scheme and made a will. A retirement budget should have been developed. Interests, hobbies and activities should also be considered and the establishment and practice of positive health behaviours should be encouraged.

Nutrition

Older adults may experience a greater proportion of nutritional problems compared to other age groups because of an increasing incidence of disease. Generally, older adults will need a balanced diet, although they may have reduced requirements for kilojoules where there is reduced activity experienced. Special diet-related problems in old age include obesity, dehydration and malnutrition.

Being old and overweight can cause various problems. It can cause damage to joints and therefore decrease mobility. It may result in the older adult experiencing fatigue on effort and reduce life satisfaction or even longevity. Obesity may also increase the older person's risk of falling and predispose them to Diabetes Type II.

The older adult is more vulnerable to fluid and accompanying electrolyte imbalances especially if they are unable to obtain fluid for themselves. Significant numbers of older people admitted to hospital are diagnosed with dehydration (Joanna Briggs Institute for Evidence-Based Nursing and Midwifery, 2001). Hot weather may deplete some older people of body fluids. The nurse should ensure that older people take adequate fluid and that those fluids are readily available. Water is preferable to tea and coffee as these act as diuretics.

A person is considered malnourished if the dietary intake of one or more essential nutrients (e.g. calories and protein) falls under the recommended daily intake (Miller, 2009). Older adults who are malnourished may appear well fed or even obese because they consume adequate or excessive calories which do not have very much nutritional value. Other causes of malnutrition include low-income, social isolation, alcohol abuse, missing teeth or ill fitting dentures.

Physical activity

We all know (in theory at least) that keeping a physically active lifestyle usually attracts health benefits. However, a large proportion of the population, including older adults, lives sedentary lives and does not, therefore, experience these health benefits. Health care professionals often have regular contact with older people and are thus ideally suited to promote the importance of regular physical activity. In a study by Hirvensalo, Heikkinen, Lintunen and Rantanen (2003), the researchers investigated whether advice by health care professionals (e.g. physicians, physiotherapists, public health nurses) was associated with increased exercise activity in non-institutional older people. It was discovered that their advice to exercise was strongly associated with an increase in physical exercise.

Health promotional activities have been directed toward particular groups of older adults, including those in hospital, Aboriginal older adults (see Crowe, 1996; Koori Connections: Indigenous Equity Strategies, in Health Promotions Strategies, volume 6, Number 1, February, 2006, Department of Human Services, Victorian Government) and those with a chronic illness (e.g. Richmond and McCracken, 1996).

Chapter 2

Aged Care – Setting the policy agenda for nursing and health

Professor Tracey McDonald, RN, RM, DNEd., BHA, MSc., PhD RSL LifeCare Chair of Ageing, Faculty of Health Sciences, ACU

Objectives:

This chapter will enable the reader to:

1) Demonstrate why it is essential to be aware of policy issues in relation to aged care;
2) Define the characteristics of a 'good policy';
3) Explore definitions of policy. Which one appeals to you and why?;
4) Examine the process involved in policy development;
5) Discuss why it is important to evaluate policy;
6) Describe what factors influence policy development;
7) Justify the proposition that nurses must be involved in policy development, implementation and evaluation at various levels; and

8) Identify policies that have shaped the aged care industry in Australia and New Zealand.

Awareness of policy in our lives

For many of us our first introduction to policy issues is likely to occur through the media as part of a newsworthy story that relates to some statement of policy which has been found ether to have been wanting in some way or perhaps has not been adhered to. During the lead-up to a government election contenders are often asked to declare their policies on certain topics such as provision or services for particular groups, or how funding could be allocated to emphasise a policy priority area or to preserve a service or location of interest.

In an employment context, policy is something set down by employers and managers to guide the organisation's approach to providing a service or dealing with anticipated events such as fire evacuation. Policies are usually accompanied by procedures and, for the more critical of these, training is provided for all staff who may have to become involved in implementing the procedure. Employers also follow policy obligations placed upon them through legislation that covers their industry and these obligations commonly form the basis upon which organisational policy is developed and implemented.

Health policy abounds across society and can be detected in healthy living campaigns that attempt to dissuade people from smoking tobacco or abusing alcohol and other drugs. Recently the health-reducing effects of obesity have been the subject of public education campaigns through television, radio and the print media in Australia. By placing the issue and consequences of not dealing with it before the general public, perceptions of the significance of the problem are influenced and result in changes to the way people regard health and ill-health, as well as their role in managing their own health. As in many advanced economies, Australia's current population is more highly educated and health-conscious than any previous generation and as a result the public is able to make decisions about personal health, risks associated with lifestyle choices and the services that may be needed.

At the heart of any policy platform is government policy which emerges from quite complex and often convoluted policy-making processes. Understanding these processes requires an appreciation of the theoretical frameworks, the institutional authority, the types of information used, the values and motivations of the policymakers and the political, professional and industrial contexts in which the processes occur.

'Good' policy is that which generates the outcomes or consequences it is intended to achieve. Producing 'good' policy requires that the policy be developed by people who have the authority to do so; the policy must set out a plan for action that is feasible – that is, it is achievable in terms of time or resources – and that it has the support of the people who will be most affected by the policy if it is implemented. When we hear of 'failed' policy it is usually in relation to a failure of one of these requirements. For instance, a policy may be developed by highly qualified people with legitimate authority but fails because the resources are simply not available to thoroughly implement it, or people find that the effects of the policy are different or worse than expected and so there is an outcry to have the policy removed or reviewed. Such unintended consequences may be found only at the time of policy implementation. However, such an outcome reflects poorly on the policy-makers involved and their approach towards policy formulation. It is worthwhile to reflect on the possibility that a policy failure for some people and groups may in fact represent a policy success for others who may have worked to influence the process to their advantage.

Efforts to influence policy processes are expected to occur at all levels and stages of policy development and review. Because policy affects work and personal opportunities, we have an abiding interest in what the policy may contain, how it is interpreted by different stakeholders and how it is implemented and enforced. By knowing how policy can be linked to resources and the rules it may contain governing access to funding, one can gain a competitive advantage over others who may be less aware of the policy and its contents. Once a policy is developed, there is usually some pathway to resources, opportunities or funding for those deemed eligible under the policy. For instance, if a particular issue is accepted as a national priority area, funding becomes available for targeted research, service development, training and education and the formation of partnerships that previously may not have been possible to set up or sustain.

Policies can be quite focused, especially if they pertain to an essential service or the protection of vulnerable people. The aged care industry is such an example. Policy interests held by government, service providers, clients and the general public and civil organisations such as trade unions and advocacy groups all revolve around the provision of an essential service; employing competent people and maintaining a sustainable industry. Quality aged care services depend on a policy environment that enables service operators to provide expertise and function successfully.

What is policy?

The word 'policy' is used in a multitude of ways to refer to aspects of the policy process. Gardiner (1992:6) recommends the categorisation used by Hogwood and Gunn (1989: 13-19) to describe the uses of the term:

- A broad label to describe a particular field of activity (e.g. welfare policy).
- An expression of general purpose or desired state of affairs (e.g. the Madrid International Plan of

Action on Ageing developed by the United Nations in 2002).

- Specific proposals contained in government plans (e.g. plans for programs to be developed to support international policies or declarations).
- Decisions of government that together constitute a pattern of related decisions which can be regarded as a policy (e.g. separate Federal Government decisions in 1990 to limit fees paid to aged care providers while increasing regulatory control over standards were described as a deliberate policy by the government even though it was not an announced policy).
- A program established by the government (e.g. Northern Territory intervention into child health and safety issues in 2007).
- Output, or what the government actually delivers compared with what it promises to deliver (e.g. funding or human resources promised, or a particular approach agreed upon). Outputs can also be the level of expenditure by a government although this is a simplistic approach to valuing a policy.
- Outcome, or what is actually achieved by the actions of governments. Outcomes can be the results of expenditure measured in non-monetary terms such as general health outcomes, which is a more sophisticated way to value a policy and is an approach that appeals to those who hope to benefit from the implemented policy.

Policy development and implementation

Policy development can be described as a series of stages. However, in reality the process can commence at any point and refer back and forth across all tasks. For the purposes of discussion the tasks that need to be accomplished include:

1. Problem identification

Involvement of the general public has become part of the process of problem identification, often through television, radio and other media. The goal is to create a groundswell of support or sympathy that increases the importance of the problem and therefore the chance of it receiving attention from policymakers. In 2009 the media in Australia exerts considerable pressure on government Ministers and departments to respond quickly to instances of personal disadvantage. By sensationalising the issue, the media has shown that it can generate a response from the highest level of political standing in this country despite the danger that ministerial responses may be mistaken as policy statements.

Civil organisations such as special interest and advocacy groups, trade unions and social movements can also raise issues that can be the start of policy review or development. In this way, civil groups can transfer what may be a personal problem to the status of a social problem. For instance, the feminist movement of the 1970s, the disability movement of the 1980s and the gay liberation movement or the 1990s successfully raised social awareness of their issues resulting in policy being developed to address many of their concerns through legislation.

More and more frequently, issues and problems are identified through research conducted by universities or industry groups and then used as a basis for informing the general public and the government. While research is not always required to substantiate policy activities, it does appear to garner more support than the recounting of a tale of misery or loss in order to gain support. Often the research is conducted on issues that are not directly concerned with policy. However, the implications of the findings may well be of interest to policy makers if the impact on technology, the workforce, public safety, disease prevention or treatment efficacy is significant.

The benefits of research as a basis for problem identification are that the scope and implications of the problem can be made known along with possible causes and recommendations for action. The danger of relying on one incident as a justification to build or review public policy lies in the possibility of endorsing 'bad' policy. That is, that the policy response is unjustified, that it is perhaps not feasible in its application across many people who were not involved in the incident, and the outcry from those who believe they should not be further regulated on the basis of an incident that may or may not reoccur.

2. Policy formulation

Participatory democracy is said to allow for openness and transparency in government and, in the area of policy development, it allows for many interest group and stakeholders to express their views. This is essentially a pluralist approach to policy development and is considered the ideal to which most policymakers aspire. It requires a mechanism whereby different voices can be heard on the issue in an environment of equity and respect. Usually experts and stakeholder groups are invited to participate in a 'reference group' which is asked to examine the issues and recommend policy strategies that may resolve them. The group is managed by the government, usually public servants from the department that will develop and implement the policy, and the group will disband once the policy is developed. In some instances the group may be asked to continue to oversee implementation as an expert group able to recommend changes as needed. Industry consultation is a crucial part of the policy formulation process in that the issue of intended and unintended consequences can be analysed and changes made or amelioration strategies adopted to avoid a 'failed' policy.

3. Policy adoption

The policy proposal is prepared by the public service using formal language or similarly clear terminology and sent to the Minister for the government department responsible for the policy. At this stage the Minister may wish to test the policy in terms of public reaction or merit before approving it. If the policy requires legislative changes it will be scheduled for parliamentary debate unless enabling legislation is in place to allow public servants and the Minister to enact sub-legislation or regulations. When given legal authority, the policy is legitimate and can be used as a basis for action to deal with the problem or issues it was developed to address.

4. Policy implementation

Policy is often trialled or modelled during a transition phase prior to implementation in order to estimate its impact or to detect any unforeseen problems. It is then scheduled for implementation on a specified date. Those affected by the policy are usually provided with information and sometimes training or resources to up-skill prior to the introduction of any policy that will cause changes to their industry. For example, changes to the way the aged care industry is funded were implemented in March 2009. Prior to implementation, pilot programs were used in various regions of Australia to test whether the desired outcomes and outputs were being achieved. Industry training was provided by the government to ensure that aged care providers and their key staff were aware of the changes and had the skills and understanding to work within the new system of funding. The reference group was retained as an advisory committee upon the implementation of the new policy.

National policies may need to be implemented by state governments, each of which has its own legislature and responsibilities and, invariably, their own state priorities for expenditure and policy development. The State-Federal fiscal relationship is key to the uptake by states of national policy directives. Various arrangements around funding exist, such as the Medicare and Goods and Services Tax agreements, which are negotiated between state and federal governments. Where agreement exists on joint policy goals the policy is more likely to be implemented without delay. Part of this implementation process could be the development of state policy frameworks to enable regional issues and contexts to be considered and catered for in the policy. Where there is no agreement, or where funding incentives are used to make an unpalatable policy more acceptable, delays in policy implementation can seem inevitable.

5. *Policy evaluation*

Once implemented, policies need to be evaluated in order for us to understand the outcomes and outputs involved. Evaluation against the intended outcomes for the target population is often subsumed under an evaluation of the outputs or expenditure on the program. Part of the issue is that such evaluations can be expensive and the government may not be inclined to undertake an evaluation that may cast doubts on what appears to be a successful policy. For some programs, a review date is set early in the process of policy development so that the costs associated with evaluation are incorporated in the project planning. Government evaluation of policy is generally undertaken where there is some concern about its alignment with the Australian constitution, statutes and regulations, funding outputs, public service operations and priorities, political implications and whether there is an impending election.

Where evaluation is not undertaken by a government it is possible for the industry and other stakeholders to undertake an evaluation of their own. The results can then be used to lobby the government to undertake a more substantial review if necessary. For instance, an industry review of the costs associated with meeting regulatory compliance under the residential aged care industry Resident Classification Scheme funding arrangements was undertaken in 2005 by the Aged Care Association Australia. The report revealed that an estimated $142,000,000.00 per annum was being spent by the industry on activities solely associated with compliance with government regulations around funding. The Aged Care Association Australia report was made available to the government and others and has since been referred to in several policy discussions related to strategies introduced in 2009 for reducing 'red tape' within the funding system for aged care.

The types of outcomes that can prompt non-government actors to undertake policy evaluation include concerns by interest groups about the economic impact of the policy on scarce resources, or how it affects other activities that they regard as priorities. There can also be concerns about cultural protection where policies appear to undermine or conflict with traditions or values held by particular groups or communities.

Influencing policy

Policy is inherently political because of competing interests among all stakeholders involved in what is otherwise touted as a rational process. Politics is related to the wielding of power, and the eventual result of that influence can be policy. Political activity is not restricted to government committees, nor is it to be dismissed as a possibility. Political behaviour, even in the workplace, can influence the development of policies that enable decision-making to occur and productivity to increase.

Professional groups are well-known to be politically active in achieving the types of policies that can advantage their members. The medical profession has been particularly successful in influencing health, insurance, research and other policies that continue to support their central position within the health professions.

Political action usually involves activities that lead to the acquisition, development or use of influence over others and resources in order to achieve some desired outcome. Political action is particularly effective where there is uncertainty within the organisational or professional environment and where there is disagreement about available options and possibilities. In this way political action can be constructive in combining rational argument and influence over decisions that will reduce organisational uncertainty. It could even be said that politics provides the incentive and the means some people need to achieve goals within an organisation. For instance, uncertainty in organisational policies can arise from structural changes such as changes in procedures, time-frames or role responsibilities. When work relationships are altered through changes in scope or introduction of technology or new work categories, power and influence are shifted. Skills and abilities thought to be valuable under the previous system (e.g. teaching) may be devalued under a new system that values only funded research, leaving those with expertise in teaching politically vulnerable, that is, unless they engage in strategic activity to increase their power in some other way, such as getting themselves onto a policymaking committee.

Nurses and politics

Nurses are the largest group of health care professionals, yet politically they are relatively powerless in Australia. This is in spite of the versatility and range of skills and knowledge that enable nurses to locate people within situations of risk and help them to rally their own resources to be able to either resolve the problem or adapt in a healthy way to the situation.

The story of politics in nursing usually relates to internal, intraprofessional conflicts or industrial contests with employers. Nurses who transcend these limitations and move into legal, managerial, political and other fields of influence can experience a disconnection with nurses who remain in clinical roles and others who decry the accumulation and use of power. Whether nurses who achieve positions of power exercise it to the advantage of the nursing profession is not known, although there has been some professional advancement of nurses through their involvement in the development of government policy around professional education. As with other professions, nurses would benefit from partnerships with nursing and non-nursing colleagues, or by forming coalitions that create power and influence the policy that governs their access to education, workplaces, funding and their status in society.

Through an understanding of policy, nurses and others can come to appreciate that the underlying principle in policy formulation is 'control'. This can include control of workers, of members of organisations, of situations and of resources. In the organisational sense it can even determine which priorities are to be established and followed by nurses who, through their employment contract, are obliged to adhere to the organisational policies of their employer. Policies that guide and even bind nursing practice arise through a process of policy formulation which would be more politically effective if it were initiated by nurses rather than waiting to respond to policies made by others.

Aged care and the policy agenda in Australia

Prior to 1967 aged care in nursing homes was regulated and overseen by state governments. Earlier services for the aged from the early 1950s included convalescent homes, rest homes and some boarding houses where very little regulation applied in terms of standards of safety and quality. Government had minimal involvement with what were privately owned services conducting their business as they saw fit.

The *National Health Act 1953,* under the jurisdiction of the Commonwealth Department of Health, brought oversight to the private sector, while the following year the *Aged and Disabled Persons' Homes Act 1954* brought non-profit aged care providers under the jurisdiction of the Department of Social Services. During the period between 1953 and 1973 privately owned convalescent homes received a subsidy for each patient and a monitoring system was introduced to count the number of patients. Social Services provided financial support to Older Person's Hostels to supplement the rent.

From 1973 to 1987 several policy initiatives occurred that affected the nature and number of aged care service providers. January 1973 saw the first 'benefit' system introduced for nursing homes, and to be eligible, nursing home providers had to have registered by 31 December 1972. This scheme was voluntary a result of the policy that set up the Participating Scheme. This scheme, under the *Nursing Homes Assistance Act 1974,* subsidised providers for 'costs necessarily incurred' in delivering ordinary care and extensive care to older people residing in nursing homes. This scheme was reviewed and refined in October 1977. However, throughout this period there were growing concerns about the cost of the program, despite the number of people able to receive the subsidy being restricted to a planning formula that allowed for 70 out of every 1,000 people aged 70 years or over to access nursing home care.

In July 1987 standard costing was introduced to make provision for non-professional care costs. This method was known as the Standard Aggregate Module, or SAM. The planning formula was changed to allow 40 out of every 1,000 people aged 70 years or over to access nursing home care and 60 out of every 1,000 people aged 70 years and over to access hostel care. The following year a policy change allowed for the introduction of the costing of nursing and professional care under the Care Aggregated Module, or CAM, and in NSW the introduction of the *Nursing Homes Act NSW (1988).* Nurses in management positions were immediately and irreversibly moved into financial and business management roles in addition to their professional leadership roles.

Under the new policy nurse managers were required to reconcile CAM funding and expenditure and manage nursing homes with five categories of residents under the Resident Classification Index or RCI introduced in 1988. Hostels had three categories of residents funded under the PCAI. This period also saw the introduction of 'entry contributions', now referred to as bonds, and the first concessional residents drawn from less fortunate situations were admitted for care.

During the decade 1987 to 1997 significant policy development occurred for the aged care industry and all who worked within it. Of particular interest was the emergence of the notion of residents' rights and responsibilities which was announced in a charter within aged care policy. Along with this were several reviews: the CAM Review (1987), Living in a Nursing Home (1988), Gazette S303 (1987), which outlined the proposed new service inspection policy, the Practical Guide to Duty of Care (1988), the Review of Documentation and Accountability (1993), Continuity of Care and community care pilot programs (1993-95). The cost of expanding and improving aged care services was also increasing and the Commonwealth Own Purpose Outlays (COPO) funding was initiated in 1993 and indexed to other economic indicators.

The *Aged Care Act 1997* and Quality Principles brought to the aged care industry a comprehensive regulatory framework that introduced several key policies: COPO would remain as an indexation system; 'ageing in place' would apply to residents in all contexts to prevent them being moved when their condition changed; accommodation bonds were applied to all levels of care (high and low care). However, in response to effective lobbying from senior groups in the community, the Prime Minister removed the option of bonds from high care and replaced it with an accommodation charge.

The funding of residents and their care was changed to the Resident Classification Scheme (RCS) and was based on proof that appropriate care had been delivered. Residents were classified under eight levels, Level 8 being a social care category with no funding. Levels 1 to 4 were considered to be high care and Levels 5 to 8 low care. Procedures for changing the category of care for individual residents were part of the policy and every resident needed to be fully assessed each year against 20 questions for funding to continue. Claims for increased levels of care and funding were validated by Commonwealth nursing officers who visited aged care homes and rigorously reassessed the claims, either confirming or downgrading them. If downgrading occurred a penalty of six month's retrospective funding for that person was levied against the home.

The *Aged Care Act 1997* removed the need for acquittal (reconciliation of expenditure for care services) and replaced it with a system of accountability for outcomes rather than process. The new system of mandatory accreditation by the Australian Aged Care Standards and Accreditation Agency (the Agency) and the Complaints Resolution Scheme (CRS) shifted the focus from effort to results. Accreditation focuses on quality outcomes measured against 44 outcomes within four standards: management, care, lifestyle and environment. Homes found non-compliant are placed on a timeline for improvement plus increased scrutiny. Where the non-compliance poses a threat to residents, the home is sanctioned and funding reduced. The CRS, along with subsequent iterations leading to the current Complaints Investigation Scheme (CIS), is available to all clients, families and concerned others who wish to raise complaints about resident care. The CRS/CIS accepts anonymous complaints and investigates them rigorously, often referring matters to the Detailed Assessment Team (DAT) and to the Agency for further scrutiny.

Substantial growth occurred during 1987 to 1997, particularly in the non-profit sector, which has tax-exempt status to enable a focus on serving those less fortunate. To ensure that the growth of the non-profit sector remained within feasible bounds, access to residential aged care became subject to assessment by the Aged Care Assessment Teams (ACAT) based in public hospitals and partially funded by the Federal Government. These teams of medical, nursing and allied health practitioners continue to control eligibility for aged care services and thereby the rate of growth within the industry.

Other regulatory frameworks associated with the *Aged Care Act 1997* include building certification, to ensure the environment is safe for all, the Aged Care Principles that spell out in detail all aspects of regulatory compliance imposed and Aged Care Agreements (containing the Charter of Residents Rights and Responsibilities) between service providers and service recipients.

Since 1997 there has been a growth of community-based aged care through the Community Aged Care Packages (CACP), which are funded as low care, non-nursing services to people in their homes, and the Extended Aged Care at Home (EACH) packages, which fund nursing care for people at home. Transitional care funding has also been made available to hospitals to allow for a defined period of rehabilitation to occur for older persons within hospitals.

Changes have also occurred with the aged care bed planning formula which in 2009 was as follows: 44 high care +44 low care +25 community care places for every 1,000 Australians aged 70 years and over. These substantial changes to aged care services placed a strain on the COPO indexation arrangements and in 2004 the Conditional Adjustment Payment (CAP) was introduced to increase funding for services that met certain reporting requirements. Services which benefited include staff education, annual auditing and publishing of accounts and participation in government-initiated workforce surveys.

Several policy reviews have occurred since 1997, including the Two-Year Review of Aged Care released in 2001 and the Aged Care Pricing Review (2004), which examined the sustainability of aged care services under the funding and regulatory systems managed by the Department of Health and Ageing. In NSW the *Nursing Homes Act 1998* was repealed, resulting in national consistency under the Aged Care Act for industry regulation. As a result of these reviews and lobbying from aged care peak organisations and civil organisations, a process of review was initiated concerning the RCS funding system and associated policies.

From 2003 to 2009 a detailed review of the residential aged care funding policy occurred and the policy was introduced to the residential aged care sector in March 2009. The major difference between this policy and the RCS is the shift of emphasis from proving through documentation that care did occur with annual applications for continued funding, to assessing residents for anticipated care needs under the Aged Care Funding Instrument (ACFI), with no annual reassessments. Application for changes to ACFI can be made should the person's condition change and validation of the claims is linked to the origin of the admission. If admitted to residential care from hospital, the claim is validated within six months to determine if significant change has occurred since the acute hospital episode. This new system of funding is more complex than the RCS, which had seven funded categories plus supplements and 64 possible outcomes. In the interest of ensuring that aged care services are not disadvantaged during the introductory phase of ACFI, existing residents will remain on the equivalent RCS funding level (known as 'grand-parenting') until an application is made by the service provider to claim under the new ACFI system. It is anticipated that by 2011 all residents will be funded under the ACFI policy and limits placed by the Department of Health and Ageing on the top funding categories will be lifted.

Aged care and development of quality standards in New Zealand

Residential aged care in New Zealand shares many of the core principles of service and quality care with those embraced by Australia. Both countries focus on the outcomes of services for both residents and their organisations and both are confronted with shortages of skilled staff and increases in acuity of people seeking to access care services. Key differences exist in relation to how the service sector is structured and funded, and how accreditation is achieved.

New Zealand aged care is a responsibility shared between 21 District Health Boards (DHB) which work with aged services providers, including not-for-profit trusts (around 25% of all service providers), to provide rest home and other geriatric services. In this way all of aged care is essentially privatised (that is, not government-owned) even though government subsidy is paid as part of the contract for services. The market in New Zealand is much less restricted that in Australia, owing to the limited formal restrictions placed on the things for which residents can be charged and the diversity of services that can be provided. For instance, residents wanting to access more salubrious accommodation and hotel services (premium accommodation) can be charged what the market will bear which is different from Australia where these charges are closely regulated under the Extra Service provisions of the *Aged Care Act 1997.*

The development of Quality Health Accreditation in New Zealand has involved iterative changes to the quality health standards over many years. The initial focus of the standards was on organisational structures and the processes in which departments and professional services were involved. In 1995 a significant review of standards moved the emphasis of health care to be more focused on clients and community needs, client rights and cultural appropriateness. At this time consumer issues were acknowledged and incorporated into the standards. For instance consumers were concerned about their opportunities to participate in decision-making and service delivery, access to information about services and service planning, giving feedback on services and participating in resolving any problems and issues raised. The revised standards were released in 1997 and achieved a more streamlined system of quality and safety requirements than previously because duplication had been reduced and the emphasis moved more to outcomes than inputs. Process standards and structural requirements were retained and incorporated within the assessment and care planning standard.

In 2000 the board of the New Zealand Council on Healthcare Standards undertook extensive work on developing the standards and systems for auditing and implementing change. A major aspect of this change was a move to a model of full client-focused continuum of care. Several standards were trialled with the continuum of care model, beginning with hospice, primary care and mental health modules. Within four years the full continuum across all standards was achieved and implementation occurred in 2001. Nine months later a revised version of the standards was issued by the newly named Quality Health New Zealand, and this included new and revised sector standards, more streamlining and a refinement and clarification of the standards in response to client and surveyor feedback. At this point sector-specific standards modules were developed as well.

The reviews between 1995 and 2000 culminated in the *Health and Disability Services (Safety) Act 2001* which, among many other changes, moved service licensing to certification against the much refined and tested care standards. The most significant of these care standards is NZ8134, which covers infection control, patient restraint minimisation and from 2009 also included a mental health care standard for quality and safety.

Compliance with care standards is required for certification to be achieved or retained and this of course requires auditors to examine the operations of service providers. Services needing to be certified under the Health and Disability Services (Safety) Act apply to the Ministry of Health, and as part of this application auditors will nominate which DAA they will use and, of course, pay a fee. The surveyors (auditors) then begin to assist the service to prepare through self-audits on the essential standards of NZS 8134:2001, NZS 8142:2000 and NZS 8141:2001, plus a tool for NZS 8143:2001 for mental health services. Usually the auditing team will provide on-site feedback to the service managers about any issues in meeting the standards. When all standards have been met, the auditors will report to the Ministry of Health, where certification is decided.

New Zealand has three groups of auditors who could be involved at any time in ensuring that service providers are compliant with regulation and contractual obligations.

The first group is made up of external, independent auditors designated by the Director General of Health to monitor the standards using an outcomes focus. These designated audit agencies (DAA), currently comprising five organisations across New Zealand, are available for selection by service providers and, equally, service providers can cancel their service and engage another company if they choose. The DAA auditor then audits against a standard template which measures attainment of the care standard on a four-level grading system. If an aspect of a standard is not attained the DAA auditor will estimate the risks associated with this non-compliance and include that estimate in the report which goes to the Ministry. The Ministry staff then certifies the audited service for a period ranging from six months to four years. Criteria for deciding the length of accreditation have only recently been available to the aged care industry.

The second group of auditors are part of the District Health Boards with which services providers work to provide aged care services. These DHB auditors are mandatory, meaning that service providers have no choice of auditor and no mechanism for negotiating the timing or person involved. The major issue is that DHB auditors can and do second-guess the DAA auditors, causing considerable uncertainty within the industry along with political competition between the two groups of auditors. There are moves afoot to merge both regulatory and contract auditing functions and a major review in 2009-2010 will include systems for ensuring safety and quality as well as the provision of adequate aged care services to meet the future requirements of an ageing population. What does not appear to be included is research on the effectiveness of audited services on improving safety and quality.

The third group of auditors can involve any of the above groups or another independent researcher engaged to investigate an issue that has attracted public attention, usually through the news media or questions to the Minister. An example would be the rarely-occurring instance of elder abuse covered by the media and causing the Minister to seek more detailed information.

Nursing and aged care

From the previous section it is clear that the aged care industries in both Australia and New Zealand have experienced immense changes in policy since the middle of last century. These policy changes have increased in speed and intensity during the past decade and there is no indication that policy development will stall in the foreseeable future. Nurses working within this environment have been required to adapt and work with the many changes in practice driven by these new policies. Primarily the industry has established itself as a central, essential service to society, and in order to deliver safe and effective aged care it requires a range of competent and professional employees and managers capable of performing well in this fully accountable system of social and nursing care.

Nurses are pivotal to the delivery of aged care services and therefore the industry has a keen interest in nurse education, regulation and its ongoing development. In Australia changes in service eligibility policy under ACFI are resulting in more admissions of people with a need for complex care, including rehabilitation, palliation, psychogeriatric care, sub-acute medical conditions and community care. Similar patterns of demand are occurring in New Zealand. Clinical practice in aged care therefore bears little resemblance to nursing roles in the rest homes of yesteryear. Clinical leadership, team management, quality management, multidisciplinary collaboration, service marketing, client liaison, environment and financial management are all part of the registered nurse's role and, increasingly, endorsed enrolled nurses are joining in these tasks.

Because of the increasing acuity of residents it is essential that aged care services and local hospitals have a productive working partnership built upon mutual professional respect. Aged care and the public health sector are becoming more closely linked as our population ages, and this offers opportunities for development partnerships and research projects around the care of older people. A major aspect of these links is the influence that aged care has over policy affecting the acute hospital system and how it manages and treats older people transferring to and from residential care.

Nurse education

Nurse education in Australia has undergone significant change since the mid 1960s when the apprenticeship model was in use and located within hospitals. Much of the change in nurse education has been led by policy changes initiated by lobbying from nurses for access to professional level education. The putsch for transferring nurse education from hospitals to tertiary education relied on the assumption that it would lead to greater individual growth, enabling nurses to approach professional communication, problems and decisions with a higher level of intellectual competence. It was also widely believed that nurses educated in this way would have enhanced employment prospects in a greater variety of practice contexts.

Nursing in Australia led the charge to establish beginning competencies for professional practice. The impetus for this concerted effort was in part a response to the widespread criticism of nursing organisations that had successfully altered the basic educational requirements for nursing. Consumers, social groups, other professions, employers and many senior nurses criticised the transfer of nurse education to colleges of advanced education. Graduate nursing competence was often questioned and nurse registering authorities were asked to explain why graduates were not as competent as previous hospital graduates had been. This furore took a toll on the status and stability of nursing as a legitimate profession and a sharp decline in applicants to nursing programs occurred. Graduate registered nursing numbers fell by 20% over five years and various other professional groups and employers pointed to workforce shortages to justify calls for a return to hospital-based programs. These politically effective strategies directly challenged professional nursing groups on their ability to exercise control over nurse education and practice. In other words, political antagonists claimed that nursing did not possess the capacity for professional cohesiveness, nor did they possess the ability to self-regulate, both key characteristics of a profession.

In an effort to reassure the general public and other professional groups that this new system of pre-registration education would produce safe nurses, the Australian Nursing Council Incorporated (ANCI) undertook a national consultancy to develop National Competencies for RNs and ENs in recommended domains (Gray, 1993). The competency statements were used to guide curricula development across various higher education institutions hoping to license their programs with the state nurse registering authorities, as well as clarifying to the general public what nurses do and what standards could reasonably be expected of a beginning nurse.

The point to be made with regard to policy is that nursing developments were prompted by concerns expressed in the media and in other forums about public safety issues that could arise because nurses were being prepared differently from the hospital training system which had been shown for many decades to be adequate. The motivations behind these expressions of concern can only be speculated upon. However, there is little doubt that some were motivated by political and competitive interests that would benefit from continuing constraints upon nurse education and authority in order to extend their scope of practice. As a result, nursing sought to establish professional credibility through regulation of entry and assurances of scrupulous practice by the establishment of a code of ethics. Further development of education opportunities that could support professional specialisation was a strategy hoped to be successful in increasing access to resources and extending the professional power base of nursing.

The transition to higher education was hampered by nursing traditionalists with a tendency to cling to past models of practice and didactic teaching approaches, and this did little to prompt the development of the hoped-for personal attributes of higher education graduates. Others sought to copy medical education approaches and centralised natural sciences in their curriculum, as well as emphasising hospital practice. This has been detrimental to the development of student appreciation of other practice settings such as community, aged care, mental health and disability nursing. As part of the effort to establish a discipline of nursing, the focus was shifted more and more to positivist theories which did little to encourage students in social and community engagement or to prompt them to consider how to influence the societies and values that impact on their professional and personal lives.

Enrolled nursing

Currently, professional registration is set up to control the education and practice standards of registered and enrolled nurses as well as more advanced professional groups such as nurse practitioners and midwives. While the purpose of regulation through a system of licensing is to assure the public that licensed practitioners are safe, because of their education and accountability, the status derived from having professional registration is much sought-after by those who are not required to have a license to practice. Nursing traditionalists hold that only those who are registered or enrolled can be considered 'nurses', while those who undertake nursing work are not.

In terms of policy change, it is worth remembering that nurse aides were introduced early last century to the hospital workforce so that they could assist registered nurses or 'sisters' in their work. Registered nurses delegated increasingly complex tasks to nurse aides, and because these delegations might entail risks to safety it was considered worthwhile to set up a system whereby registration authorities could impose regulatory accountability upon them. Enrolled nurses have further developed their skills and scope of practice, and now consider a career as an enrolled nurse to be an end in itself. Of course, a pathway to registered nurse education has always maintained a formal linkage between these two licensed groups of nurses.

Enrolled nursing roles and career structures have expanded over the past few decades. However, the relationship between enrolled and registered nursing has placed restrictions on the former through policies insisting that enrolled nurses may only practice under the supervision of registered nurses. Nursing policies such as this may have been developed to protect patients in acute hospital settings, but an unintended consequence is the undermining of employment and practice opportunities that would become available to enrolled nurses wishing to work in non-hospital environments.

In aged care contexts, policy restrictions placed on enrolled nurses by registered nursing bodies has so constrained their scope of practice and employment options as to render enrolled nurses uncompetitive, with unlicensed workers performing similar nursing work. The burgeoning of care workers within the context of community, aged and disability services has been supported by the development of nationally accredited education programs under the Australian Qualifications Framework (AQF). Enrolled nurse qualifications are now included in the AQF along with a range of other industry qualifications of the same standing.

The policy arena for the nursing profession is again being pressured as we debate issues around acknowledging care workers as nurses and whether these workers need to be licensed as a matter of public (and professional) safety.

The aged care workforce

The bulk of aged care policy revolves around establishing a sustainable industry that employs competent people to perform an essential service to society. On this basis alone, aged care employers and managers have an interest in the education of nurses, therapists, medical practitioners, dentists and others who service clients in aged care residential and community environments. The appropriateness of health care services delivered in the aged care environment is monitored through the Aged Care Accreditation Standards as defined under the *Aged Care Act 1997.*

Nursing has traditionally been the responsibility of state governments while medicine has been a Federal Government responsibility. However, in 2009 this changed when a national registration system was introduced to cover all health professionals. Aged care is nationally regulated and, since moving into the higher education sector in the early 1990s, so too is nurse education. Nationalisation of these different aspects of health and aged care services, workforce and education has brought into focus many of the issues, canvassed above, that relate to the supply of competent professionals and other workers providing a nationally regulated service to vulnerable people.

One such issue is the diminishing supply of registered nurses for work within the aged care industry. Pressure from aged care providers is being applied to government to review the requirement for registered nurses in some aspects of aged care, simply because it is not feasible when so few registered nurses are available. Pressure from aged care providers has been instrumental in breaking down differences in state professional registration for nurses whose work in aged care takes them across state borders, where inconsistencies in registration and skill repertoire result in inefficiencies.

A major force in the setting up of the National Review of Nursing Education in 2002 was that exerted by the aged care industry in an effort to draw attention to the lack of aged care content in nursing curricula and the over-emphasis of hospital practice on undergraduate preparation. Of the 36 major recommendations from that review, 16 related directly to issues raised by aged care lobbyists. Edwards (2004) highlighted many of these issues in a subsequent report on Aged Care Core Component in Undergraduate Curricula Principles, which was to lead to increased funding to universities to support aged care components in their curricula.

In policy terms, these efforts of the aged care industry and aged care nurses has been quite successful because the policy agenda for both nursing and health needs now to include consultation with aged care services if it is to be legitimate. With the establishment of the AQF and government recognition of the difficulties facing aged care services in recruiting registered nurses, workforce solutions that maximise the use of registered nurses mean that alternative workers can be engaged to augment nursing and even substitute for nurses in some instances. Nursing in contemporary aged care contexts includes both clinical and non-clinical roles, and for nurses to maintain their core roles in this new environment they will need to adapt and respond to social and employer demands while preserving their integrity as professional nurses. Any ongoing success of nursing in aged care will depend greatly on the calibre of nurse leaders and their ability to influence the development of fresh insights by industrial and professional interest groups so that they may support change and expansion of roles embraced by aged care nurses.

Indicators of policy success

Issues raised with the government by lobby and interest groups are usually associated with the need to alter existing policy because of unintended consequences, to expand a policy that appears to be having a desirable outcome, or to seek resources to be allocated within the annual budget so that implementation and evaluation can occur. In 2004-2005 the Australian Government budget provided tangible evidence of the effective policy work undertaken persistently over many years by the aged care industry and professional nursing organisations. Aged care nurses, managers, service providers and peak industry associations aligned to raise issues and concerns with the government and then contributed time and resources to the development and review of policies that impacted on the industry and all associated with it. As a result the budget outcomes for that year set down an aged care agenda that will run for many years to come.

By participating in local and national policy development and review processes, nurses and other professionals accumulated further understanding of regulatory and policy frameworks, as well as the skills to influence policy as necessary. A successful budget outcome will also alter perceptions held by society and politico-professional groups about the significance of aged care. Budget outcomes that are seen to be linked to policy driven by aged care political efforts will continue to drive nursing and health agendas into a future where aged care issues receive equal emphasis.

The 2004-2005 budget changed aged care industry processes in service provision and regulatory compliance, and these changes will continue to impact on general nursing and health policy agendas. Aged care is now central to any conceptualisation of the health system, and this brings with it greater opportunity for influencing future policy on aged care, nursing and health.

Summary

Policy that generates the outcomes or consequences intended to be achieved can only be set up through processes that involve all who are affected by the policy. Producing 'good' policy requires that people who have the authority to make policy are involved and have the skills to determine whether the policy is feasible, that is, whether it is achievable in terms of time or resources. Importantly, the people who will be most affected by the policy if implemented must have an opportunity to participate in its development and come to support it.

Aged care has established itself as a central, essential service to society and the industry requires a range of competent people to deliver safe and effective care. Nurses are pivotal to the delivery of aged care services and the aged care industry has taken an interest in nurse education, regulation and ongoing development. As our population ages, aged care and the public health sector are becoming more closely linked, and this opens up opportunities for partnerships and projects that will improve standards and services overall.

Through the processes outlined above, the aged care industry has influenced policy affecting nursing and health and will continue to maintain positive links across the health and education systems to ensure an adequate supply of competent people to undertake nursing work in all sectors. Professional nursing needs to remain closely involved with these policy review processes to ensure an ongoing core role in aged care.

Chapter 3

Psychology of ageing

Professor Kate Moore, BA, Grad. DipAppPsych, MSc., GradDipClinMentalHlth (Hypnosis), PhD, MAPS, MAICD
Head, Psychology Theme, School of Health Sciences, CDU

Ruth Billany, BSc Joint Hons Zoology & Psychology, MA Psychology (endorsement in Health Psychology), Lecturer in Psychology, School of Health Sciences, Charles Darwin University (CDU)

Objectives:

This chapter will enable the reader to:

1) Examine Erikson's 8th stage of development. Are there later stages that he doesn't identify?;
2) Explore the proposition that older adults experience fewer life events than younger people;
3) Demonstrate an understanding of the differences between grief and depression;
4) Identify and discuss the advantages associated with old age;
5) Describe the advantages associated with volunteerism; and

6) Explore how older adults think about their ageing.

Introduction

Age and the meaning of old age have changed dramatically over the past century. In Australia, the average life expectancy of males born in 1901 was 55.2 years while for those born in 2002 it is 78.5 years. For females the figure increased from 58.8 years to 83.3 years during the same period (Australian Bureau of Statistics (ABS), 2009). As a result, the number of people aged 65 years and above has increased significantly from 4%in 1901 to 13% in 2006 (ABS, 2009). This trend will continue as the 'Baby Boomers' (those born 1946 - 1964) age. Such longevity raises questions across many domains - economic, workforce, social and health - which include not just one's physical but also one's social and psychological wellbeing. Not only does the ageing population pose problems for governments in the provision of services, it also raises questions of how we, as individuals and a society, view and experience old age and how family and health providers care for older adults.

Developmental theorists see life as a series of stages through which we pass, from infancy to childhood, adolescence, young adulthood and mature adulthood to old and (a more recent term) old-old, but it is not just the bodily stages which are important. It is how we adapt to these psychologically which contributes to our quality of life.

Erikson's psychosocial theory of personality development

Erikson (1963) argued that just as there are bodily stages, so too are there stages of psychosocial adjustment. Each of his eight stages represent a developmental hurdle that contributes to 'healthy' progression or, if the individual is not successful in completing a stage, 'unhealthy' progression. According to Erikson, unhealthy individuals will spend their lifetime attempting to deal with the conflicts and challenges that emerge as a result of their failure to pass through an earlier stage or earlier stages (Erikson, 1963) (Table 2).

Table 2: Erikson's psychosocial theory of personality development

Ages	Stages
Infancy	Basic trust versus mistrust
1.5 – 3.5 years	Autonomy versus shame and doubt
3.5 – 5.5 years	Initiative versus guilt
5.5 – 12 years	Industry versus inferiority
Adolescence	Identity versus role confusion
Young adulthood	Intimacy versus isolation
Adulthood	Generativity versus stagnation
Maturity	Ego integrity versus despair

Infancy

Erikson's first stage occurs in infancy, where healthy children develop a sense of trust as they come to view the world as a friendly place. 'Unhealthy' infants, however, begin to see the world as hostile and develop mistrust. If infants develop trust in this stage of life, they develop a hopeful attitude about life. In his second stage, children begin to learn how to live autonomously within their environment by learning to talk, walk, eat and go to the toilet without shame. Infants who have success in this stage develop a sense of control over their thoughts, emotions and behaviours. Those who do not master this stage, or those who are ridiculed in their attempts to do so, begin to feel doubt and shame about themselves.

Childhood

Between the ages of 3.5 to 5.5 years, which is Erikson's third stage, children begin to take initiative and to assert themselves appropriately, leading to a sense of purpose. Those infants who are not able to assert themselves without it leading to conflict with others may feel guilty and struggle to take the initiative. For children aged 5.5 – 12 years, which encompasses the fourth stage, Erikson proposed that they develop either a sense of capability and industriousness in their activities, which he labeled competence, or they develop feelings of incompetence and low self-worth. Children who successfully pass through this fourth stage will experience achievements at school while children who are unsuccessful will feel that they are inadequate, believing that they function at a lower level than other children. It is unclear from Erikson's theory whether this is actual or perceived inadequacy. In fact, it can be suggested that perceived failure may be just as detrimental in its effect at all stages.

Adolescence

In adolescence, Erikson argued that individuals are trying to decide who they are and what they want from life. Adolescents try to integrate various aspects of their lives, including intellectual, social, sexual and ethical aspects. Adolescents who succeed through this stage develop a sense of self-identity while those who do not remain confused about where they are going and what they want to achieve in life. Moving beyond these years, young adulthood is a time when, according to Erikson, individuals begin to be less self-focused and seek to be committed to another person. Young adults who are successful in this stage are able to love others in an unselfish way, while those who are unsuccessful may have difficulty connecting with other people.

Adulthood

The middle adulthood stage is when adults try to be productive in many aspects of life, such as through their work and raising children. Adults either develop a sense of generativity or they stagnate during this stage. In maturity, or old age, individuals are believed to be attempting to understand their life and the choices they have made. Some older adults will have gained wisdom, while others will feel a sense of despair over the mistakes they have made.

Erikson argued that each successive developmental stage is related to some basic element in society. Therefore, the stages link not just to each other but also to the development of connections between individuals and their place in the world. From this perspective, the successful and sequential transition through the stages is important. If one stage is not met, the individual will experience conflict and challenges in later stages and may not be able to successfully resolve those stages. While there is scant empirical evidence for Erikson's theory, it does make intuitive sense and has some accord with the progression outlined in Maslow's (1954) hierarchy of needs.

Maslow's hierarchy of needs

The foundation of Maslow's hierarchy begins with the satisfaction of one's physical needs:

hunger, thirst and warmth. Once these needs are met the person can focus on security needs such as shelter and safety. Together, these physical and security needs can be considered the base elements essential to a healthy individual or, more particularly, one's physical well being. In terms of the World Health Organisation's (WHO) (1947) definition of health, satisfaction of needs at these levels would contribute to one's biological health, which clearly is a basic need across the lifespan.

The higher order needs are next and these are expressed in social terms of belongingness, love and social-esteem. This is where people feel part of a family – a society – and again reflects an essential need of all people at all times and ages. Fulfilment of these needs can be interpreted as contributing to one's social health. Self-esteem, which embraces being respected and approved of by others but also, and more importantly, one's own sense of dignity and self-regard, is next on the hierarchy of needs. Self-regard or self-esteem is important to promote positive mood, and this might also be referred to as psychological health. The achievement of these needs can lead to a sense of self-actualisation – that is, the fullest development of one's talents or aspirations – which, according to Maslow, is achieved towards the end of life.

In summation, the satisfaction of these needs can be said to represent healthy individuals who have secured their various needs and achieved a sense of self actualisation which is not dissimilar to Erikson's generativity. But what happens at older ages when the physical aspects and even one's social and belongingness needs – that is, one's physical and social health – are threatened? How do we understand the impact of these threats on psychological health? Does resolving Erikson's stages or achieving Maslow's hierarchy enable people to cope with the threats and losses which are both real and often substantial in older age?

The experience of loss in the older adult

While Kraaij, Pruymboom and Garnefski (2002) found that older people experience fewer negative life events overall than younger people, they do, conversely, experience more loss events, including those associated with declining health, loss of their work role and loss of friends and loved ones (Folkman, Lazarus, Pimley and Novacek, 1987). Those who experience such losses suffer more depressive symptoms than older adults who do not experience such losses (Katona, 1993). However, it is important to emphasise that it is our perceptions of events which influence our reactions. For instance, loss of career might mean loss of identity, loss of time structure and loss of esteem for many people while for others it will mean a chance to embrace other opportunities. How we react will depend in large part upon the circumstances but more so upon our typical coping strategies. Events are typically appraised as loss, threat or harm or benign (Lazarus and Folkman, 1984) and once this primary assessment is made, the individual then asks: 'What is the effect on or for me?' Depending upon the answer to this question, the person will respond in a typical manner – approach the problem looking for a solution, enlist others to help or avoid the issue (Moore, 2003). These coping strategies vary little across the lifespan. Therefore, where circumstances permit, the aged person will continue to use the same adaptive or maladaptive strategies of their younger days.

For more interpersonal losses, the grief and coping processes can be difficult, especially if the loss is of one's partner. Not only has the person lost their life partner they have also lost their sexual partner – something that is often ignored or not countenanced by carers or those who are younger. But Lindau, Schumm, Laumann, Levinson, O'Muircheartaigh and Waite (2007), in their large, random-sample of the sex lives of older Americans, found that even in the oldest group over half of those who stated that they were sexually active (the criterion for which was low, i.e. 'at least one episode of partnered sex within the previous 12 months') did in fact have sex at least 2 to 3 times per month. Van Baarsen (2002) found that loss of a partner lowered the survivor's sense of self-esteem, resulting in higher emotional loneliness and social loneliness; the bereaved also had perceptions of less social support. While sex is often a taboo subject for many older persons, and even younger persons are often embarrassed to raise this subject with them, clearly carers still need to be cognisant of all factors related to the person's grief.

Depression associated with grief is a common response to such loss (DSM-IV, APA, 2000). However, depression which goes beyond what might be considered a 'normal' timeframe for grief must be recognised and treated. Unfortunately, of the people in an aged hostel whom McCabe, Davison, Mellor, George, Moore and Ski (2006) assessed as depressed, only 50% had a recorded diagnosis of depression, which means that 50% of those in need were left untreated. A longitudinal study by Kraaij et al. (2002) found that recent negative events were significantly related to depressive symptoms in people age 67 years and over. However, prior depression was also strongly related to current depression. Clearly, family and carers need to be vigilant for overt signs of depression such as sleeping more, lack of volition, changes in weight and somatic symptoms. Less obviously, Kraaij, et al. found that depressed people used more rumination and catastrophising strategies in dealing with events than did the non-depressed participants, even after controlling for the effects of negative life events and prior depression. Kraaij, et al.'s findings suggest that cognitive strategies might be effective in treating depression among the elderly (Engels and Vermey, 1997), but first it is essential to identify it. Carers need to be alert for changes in mood or behaviour which might indicate depression.

Other strategies to deal with loss focus on the interplay between active interventions and the adjustment of personal goals and standards to changing resources (Brandstädter and Rothermund, 2002). In their model, attempts to avoid or diminish actual or anticipated losses by instrumental, self-corrective and compensatory activities constitute an assimilative mode of coping where the individual tries to transform a negatively evaluated situation in such a way that it conforms to his own goals and aspirations. A different way of neutralising discrepancies between actual and desired states consists of adapting goals and standards to given constraints. These accommodative processes involve a devaluation of, or disengagement from, blocked goals and a lowering of personal performance standards and aspirations. Assimilative coping occurs when people feel able to actively change the situation, somewhat similar to problem-solving coping, while accommodative processes tend to become dominant when action-outcome expectancies have been eroded through repeated unsuccessful attempts to change the situation. These processes are not dissimilar to Rotter's (1966) locus of control where people are said to have an internal or an external sense of control over their environment. Brandstädter and Rothermund found that elderly people experience life changes as less controllable; they display lower levels of active instrumental coping but more acceptance and emotion regulation. Such acceptance, if and when it occurs, might be either convenient for or frustrating to family and carers: in either case, they should be aware of and respect the rights of the older adult.

Positive experiences and 'enrichment effects'

Clearly older age is not only associated with loss and with negative effect. For many people, changes in roles are positive and can open new horizons – such as engagement in activities, whether social or artistic pursuits or volunteerism. Such engagement strategies can be employed with those who are not coping well and many aged hostels and nursing homes encourage activities with the aim of improving the welfare of their residents. This is in accord with activity theory, which suggests that participation in activities, particularly social activities, should not only provide time structure but also opportunities for social support, which is a significant contributor to a positive self-concept and a concrete strategy to alleviate depression (Lemon, Bengston and Peterson, 1972). Even productive activities such as housework (which of course can also be considered obligatory) or volunteer work may provide a sense of competence or usefulness, as well as a sense of mastery which is related to life satisfaction (Mence and Chipperfield, 1997). Other activities, such as gardening for pleasure, can have a physical component – and these too have health benefits.

Activity levels predict functional and cognitive status (Garfein and Herzog, 1995), the incidence of Alzheimer's disease (Scarmeas, Levy, Tang, Manly and Stern, 2001), physical health (Everard, Lach, Fisher and Baum, 2000) and, in some studies, survival (Lennartsson and Silverstein, 2001). Of course, activity might also be related to feelings of hope and social support, and so it is important to encourage it among the aged for their psychical, social, and psychological health.

In a special journal edition on 'enrichment effects' of mental activities on adult cognitive functioning, Hertzog, Kramer, Wilson and Lindenberger (2009) concluded that 'cognitive enrichment' – a popular topic at present, where we are all encouraged to work more puzzles and such – is not a panacea against the risk of cognitive decline and dementia. They reported that the effect for cognitive-enrichment to date is small compared to the large individual differences in cognitive functioning. Further, they stated that while physical activity can delay the onset of cognitive loss associated with dementia and normal ageing, nevertheless, an active lifestyle may not provide much protection from a wide variety of negative influences on cognitive morbidity and mortality in old age. In other words, physical activity is good for mobility, well-being and helping us maintain cognitive function and mood, but like everything else it is no guarantee.

Menec (2003) found that activity levels measured in 1990 among 1,000 people aged 67 to 95 years living in the community were related to greater happiness, better function and reduced mortality as measured six years later in 1996. Generally social and productive activities were positively related to happiness, function and mortality whereas more solitary activities (e.g. handiwork hobbies) were related only to happiness. While activity levels do decline with age, Menec (2003) found that older age was not correspondingly linked with less happiness: this might be interpreted in terms of compensatory mechanisms where older people have a sense of their life achievements, a concept akin to Erikson's generativity. These findings are generally consistent with activity theory in which Lemon, et al. (1972) proposed that both the frequency of participation in activities and the level of intimacy involved are important for life satisfaction: the more intimate the activity, the greater the life satisfaction. Hence, carers need to encourage older adults to engage in communal and family activities as it is vital to their psychological wellbeing.

Certainly one activity that might meet both these criteria is grandparenthood. In an Australian study on grand-parenting, Peterson (1999) found that only 10% of Australian grandparents were unhappy with the role, while another 10% claimed that no other role in life (including that of parent and spouse) afforded them as much satisfaction as did grandparenthood. Of course not all people have grandchildren and even if they do they might live in different locations or be part of a 'split' family. This latter can be experienced as a loss by the grandparents, which many find difficult to manage. Some people seek alternative activities and volunteer their time to various organisations such as the Red Cross, the Cancer Council, local schools and seniors clubs, to name a few.

Volunteerism is a pro-social behaviour that benefits others and is positively valued by society (Gross and McMullen, 1982), and which Mezirow (1994) reported can lead to personal growth and fulfilment. According to the Australian National Survey on voluntary work (ABS, 2001), approximately one third of Australians regularly volunteer their time and skills for the benefit of others. While women contribute slightly more time each week than do men, the likelihood of volunteering is influenced more by age. Surprisingly, the highest percentage of volunteers (40.1%) comes from those in the middle years (35-44) which might be explained by an increased level of engagement in activities which are related to involvement with their children and schools. The ABS statistics also show that 32.5% of people in the 55-64 year group, 30.3% in the 65-74 year group and 17.8% aged 75 years and over volunteer their time and services. Much literature supports the positive role of volunteerism on wellbeing (e.g. Van Willigen, 2000). 'High volunteering', that is, volunteering for two or more organisations, has no more beneficial effect on wellbeing than that reported by people who volunteered for only one organisation (Oman, Thoresen and McMahon, 1999). In fact, it might be that volunteering for too many organisations results in role overload or role strain (Musick, Herzog and House, 1999).

Morrow-Howell, Hinterlong, Rozario and Tang (2003), in a sample aged over 60 years, found 34.5% of respondents volunteered – a figure not dissimilar to that of the ABS (2001) – for an average of 71.5 hours per year, although some 25% said they volunteered for more than 160 hours per year. The maximum effect on wellbeing was at around 100 hours per year (approximately 2-3 hours per week) and higher levels were not associated with increasing gains. It is not clear what mechanisms might be at work here, although one might assume that volunteerism provides the person with a role, with activities and a sense of contribution as well as enabling social networks, which are known to be important for life satisfaction and quality of life. For older adults, volunteering might also offer new social contacts. For those who are in care, even being in charge of something small like serving the cakes or setting the tables might be a role which adds to their sense of identity and mood.

Relationships and networks

We know that one's social networks can affect a range of feelings, such as one's sense of morale, notions of self-worth and life satisfaction (Barrett, 1999), and they can also influence a range of behaviours. For example, an older person's utilisation of health and social services might be encouraged and supported by their social networks (Logan and Spitze, 1994). Social networks are the collection of interpersonal ties that people of all ages maintain in varying contexts and which may or may not be supportive, but terms 'support network' and social network' are often used. Researchers, such as Wenger (1996) have identified different types of networks: 1) family-dependent networks – small groups relying on close family members; 2) locally integrated networks – large groups, including relationships with family, friends and neighbours; 3) local self-contained networks – these tend to be small and mostly neighbour-based; 4) wider, community-focused networks – large and primarily friendship focused groups; and 5) private-restricted networks – characterised by the absence of local kin and only minimal ties with neighbours.

Clearly, as one ages and one's family circumstances change, so too will the character and structure of one's networks, but what is important is that at least some ties are maintained, and some new ones developed. In a study of people aged 55 years and over, Lee and Ishu-Kintz (1987) found that the morale of their participants increased as interactions with friends increased; this was also true to a lesser extent of interactions with neighbours. Close relations are therefore important, but they vary with marital status. Married older persons tend to have larger networks than those who are unmarried (Van Tilburg, 1995), unmarried men living alone have the smallest networks, while people in the old-old category have smaller networks than young-old (Litwin and Landau, 2000). Clearly, for some old-old people and those with physical impairments (Litwin, 2001), their networks might be restricted to their carers. For many in our ageing population from nuclear families and with few or no children of their own, their friends and carers will be their prime networks. It will be important for carers to be aware of this and endeavour to accommodate a sense of relationship in their interactions with the elderly as happiness scores are known to be predicted by older adults' social relations, even after controlling for background and health characteristics (Litwin and Landau, 2000).

Perspectives and perceptions of the older adult

But what do the aged think about old age? Connidis (1989) sampled 400 community-dwelling people age 65 years and above and asked if they liked or disliked anything about their age or about growing older. Overall, respondents did not focus on the negatives, however, three groups did emerge: those with a negative, moderate or positive view of ageing. Those holding negative views were older, in poorer health and had fewer children than those holding a positive view. The causal direction is not known, but one could argue that poorer health contributed to the despondency among at least some of the negative group. A further study by Keller, Leventhal and Larson (1989), where they conducted in-depth interviews on the ageing experience with 32 community adults aged 50 to 80 years, identified five themes: 1) ageing as a natural and gradual process without remarkable features; 2) ageing as a period of life evaluation; 3) ageing as a period of increased freedom; 4) associations with physical health difficulties or concerns about health; and 5) ageing as a period of loss, both interpersonal and job-related. These themes have both positive and negative aspects, as well as some similarities with those reported by Steverink, Westerhof, Bode and Dittmann-Kohli (2001) in their study of 4,034 Germans aged 40 to 85 years.

Steverink et al. found three dimensions of the ageing experience: 1) physical decline; 2) continuous growth; and 3) social loss. Better subjective health, higher income, less loneliness, higher education and greater hope were negatively associated with physical decline and social loss and positively associated with continuous growth. Interestingly, continuous growth was correlated with hope and with positive effect and negatively correlated with physical decline, while life satisfaction and hope were positively correlated. This last is congruent with the need for us all, no matter what age, to have hope. Hope is the light which helps people survive trauma and illness, and might be said to be the last emotion before despair. The maintenance of hope or purpose in life is therefore paramount among the aged. Hope can be fostered among the aged by planning for future events, setting targets and, depending on their functional status, by recruiting them to assist others.

Meaning in life is related to purpose in life (Crumbaugh, 1968) and to Antonovsky's (1987) 'sense of coherence', which is a person's subjective perception of the world and of his or her life in it. It is 'a global orientation ... feeling of confidence that one's internal and external environments are predictable and there is a high probability that things will work out as well as can reasonably be expected'. These feelings are clearly subjective and this is emphasised by the low correlations between sense of coherence and social support, subjective wellbeing and perceived state of health, as well as the lack of correlation with economic resources. It can be inferred from these findings that a sense of coherence is independent of others from whom we might receive support, yet it is not related to physical health or socioeconomics – clearly a positive for older adults who might have reduced social networks, poorer health and few financial resources. However, it seems to be related to Erikson's generativity and to Maslow's self-actualisation – perhaps a satisfaction with one's self and one's life. However, such a sense of self, of independence, can be a source of frustration at times for the busy carer who has limited time to discuss issues but might rather have it 'just do it this way/now.' Clearly an ability to balance between the individual needs and rights and the schedules of the carer/organisation is imperative.

Influences on a person's sense of wellbeing, meaning and value are called conditions for quality of life (QoL) and these can be further classified as intra-individual (e.g. health, functional capacity and coping mechanisms) and external conditions (e.g. environment, housing and social network), some of which can be reduced or missing for older adults. Therefore, is it true that the aged population has quality of life? Predictors of QoL include functional capacity, perceived health, good housing conditions, an active life style and good social relationships. However, the dominant predictor is mood state. Ask someone what their QoL is (0 being terrible and 10 the best it can be) and then ask their mood (0 being miserable and 10 happy) – the correlation will be strong. So what does this mean for older adults who might have experienced many losses, who might be living at home or in care and who might be functional or incapacitated?

It would seem that a positive mood is integral to wellbeing, even to QoL. How then do we promote this? Where possible this is done by encouraging engagement in physical activities, engagement with others, the provision of social supports and the acknowledgement of the person as an individual. The emphasis is on respecting their rights, and their person.

Interestingly, after his death, Erikson's wife Joan proposed a further stage to his lifespan model. She suggested that a person's autonomy, independence and control are challenged during the last years and as a consequence self-esteem and confidence will weaken. While this might be true in many areas, it is important for the individual's wellbeing to promote a perception of autonomy, to provide respect and thus contribute to the individual's psychological wellbeing. This can be a challenge for busy families and carers, but it is one we all need to meet.

Chapter 4

Normal biological ageing

Dr. Mary MacGibbon, PhD (Fac. Of Med.), BSc. (Med. Sc.)
Lecturer, School of Arts and Sciences, Australian Catholic University

Objectives

This chapter will enable the reader to:

1) Review primary concepts of human biological ageing and current research trends;
2) Discuss theories of ageing in the context of specific observations and age-modulation;
3) Describe normal human biological ageing, addressing:
    a) an overview of functional changes;
    b) cellular and histological changes; and
    c) changes within each system;
4) Explore the influences of ageing on pharmacokinetics and pharmacodynamics;
5) Describe the influences of ageing on manifestations of pathology; and
6) Discuss the cumulative effect of age changes and the interaction of psychosocial, behavioural and biological factors in ageing.

Introduction

Normal ageing affects all of us with time and independently of any specific disease. For a physical or other change in those 65 years and older to be purely due to ageing, it has generally been required to be:

1) inherent, so not due to infection or an environmental factor to which some individuals may not be exposed;
2) universal (for all humans);
3) progressive; and
4) deleterious.

However, separating the influences of pure ageing mechanisms from those of disease and the environment is difficult, especially in human studies. Investigations of 'super centenarians' cast some light onto changes occurring without specific disease, although these individuals, quite apart from a lack of factors predisposing to disease, may be genetically atypical with regard to mechanisms and rate of ageing. This chapter endeavours to present the current consensus of major concepts of ageing with a focus on significant structural and functional age changes in humans.

An overview of human ageing and current research trends

Much of the period of ageing is associated with life continuing very much as normal, certainly for a significant part of these older years, indicating that biological changes over that time are not markedly intrusive or are manageable. A net improvement in quality of life may even be experienced, with a brain enriched by a lifetime of learning and memories, by grandchildren, reading, writing, travel, certain sports and greater choice over what one does each day. Some individuals may perform at their peak in certain areas, especially in intellectual output. However, significant undesirable changes are inevitable, including a slower body response to certain physical stressors, a loss of organ reserve and an increased likelihood of disease. The higher incidence of pathology is due in part to having lived long with the accumulated effects of many influences including carcinogens, inflammation, unrepaired DNA breakages and hormones, together with the expression of those inherited components which predispose to disease but which are not lethal during the reproductive years and so are less susceptible to natural selection.

For census purposes and identifying groups in the ageing population, the categories of young (65–74), middle (75–84) and old (85 on) are often used. However, with increased age we become an increasingly diverse cohort, with some individuals strong and independent well into their eighties and some frail long before then, even without evidence of specific pathology. Also, within an individual certain systems may appear to age faster than others (for example, normal lens changes may cause marked presbyopia while kidney function remains relatively youthful), while in certain years or months ageing may appear to accelerate, such as during periods of extreme stress.

So is chronological age a good indicator of biological age? The answer appears to be both 'yes' and 'no' with chronological age being just one of several very useful guides. Other popular indicators of ageing status include measurable fitness and certain blood tests reflecting organ functioning (Crimmins et al., 2008; Nakamura and Miyao, 2007). However, some of the latter may in fact be measuring disease processes, such as the serum level of an inflammatory cytokine (a proposed biomarker of ageing), which is secreted in higher amounts by ageing cells (Burton, 2009). As stated, the nature of pure ageing is elusive. The section of this chapter addressing specific human age changes describes much of the current thinking regarding histological and other biological changes. Collectively the extent to which an individual manifests these could indicate their degree of ageing, but extensive debate continues regarding which specific measures would represent overall ageing.

Although much current research explores ageing specifically, major longitudinal human ageing studies appear to focus more on the indicators and genetic determinants of 'successful ageing' in terms of robustness, health outcomes and longevity. Recent publications, including those of the two primary longitudinal ageing research groups in the US, Duke University and the Baltimore Longitudinal Study of Ageing (BLSA), address these issues and also refer to ageing and its correlates. Some of their findings are as follows.

The Duke University research provides strong evidence that a cumulative index of health and well-being deficits, called the 'Frailty Index' (F.I.), can characterise ageing-associated processes in humans and predict death better than chronological age (Hastings et al., 2008; Kulminski et al., 2008; Kulminski, 2007). The F.I. includes approximately 40 factors, including difficulties in moving, lifting and hearing and the presence of conditions such as arthritis and hypertension. The researchers report that cross-sectional analysis of the F.I. in different age groups 'exhibits accelerated increase in this measure with age till oldest-old ages (95+), with possible deceleration thereafter'. The terms used imply that the change of rate of deficit accumulation occurs within an average individual, whereas the later apparent slowing of deterioration may result from a sub-group of 'super-centenarians' who are less prone to disease or may have 'longevity alleles' and in whom ageing may have been consistently slower.

The BLSA report has found that 'performance in mobility is a marker of health status superior to any other biomedical measure', and that 'poor lower extremity performance is a robust predictor of multiple negative health outcomes' (Ferruci, 2008). Some of the primary BLSA researchers endorse the intimate association between ageing and disease, and the influence of both genes and environment, in stating that they 'have come to the fairly simple conclusion that although genes affect ageing and longevity the quality of our own ageing is strongly affected by well-known regimens, such as watching our weight and waist, eating a healthy diet, exercising regularly and maintaining an active role in society' (Ferruci, 2008). In a recent review of 'exceptional survivors' major features explored included risk factors of metabolic syndrome[1] and related processes (Willcox et al., 2008). Predictors of survival included serum levels of high-density lipoproteins (HDLs) as well as a set of novel risk factors linked to adipose-endocrine function and the insulin-like growth factor-1 axis. The report states that a growing literature suggests

---

1 Metabolic syndrome predisposes an individual to type 2 diabetes, coronary heart disease and other disorders related to plaque formation in artery walls (e.g. stroke and peripheral vascular disease), and is identified by the American Heart Association and other institutions as presence of three or more of the following risk factors: in waist circumference, triglycerides, blood pressure, or fasting glucose, or- in HDL.

genetic factors, such as a particular CETP (cholesteryl ester transfer protein) gene variant affecting HDL levels, were predictive of healthy ageing and longevity. In one group baseline physiological reserve and present health and function were the strongest survival predictors.

Theories of ageing and implications for age modulation

The processes thought to underlie the phenomenon of ageing involve two major mechanisms: (i) genetic programming, and (ii) the influences of random events, commonly termed 'stochastic'. These two mechanisms are not mutually exclusive, and an overview of current theories and supporting studies indicates that ageing is an outcome of both. When comparing mammalian species a rough inverse correlation is found between lifespan (the maximum time an individual in a species is thought to be able to live) and the basal metabolic rate, although certain variables and influences, including brain weight and regimens such as dietary restriction, can modify this relationship (Austad, 2001). Human metabolic rate and the associated mitochondrial function are to a large degree genetically determined, but by-products of normal metabolism, including reactive oxygen species such as free radicals, oxidise and damage important molecules, such as DNA, in a random fashion. Much research in gerontology explores these mechanisms and their effects, as well as molecules or regimens which increase or retard these processes (Meydani, 1999).

That we are comparable to ticking time bombs, genetically programmed to age and die, is indicated not only by the limited number of times which certain cells can divide (Hayflick and Moorhead, 1961) and our apparently finite lifespan of around 120 years regardless of environmental factors, but also by certain chromosomal disorders such as progeria and Down syndrome, which accelerate ageing, and by findings such as that of a single gene change in related, if simpler, animals and worms, which can extend lifespan five-fold (Lakowski and Hekimi, 1996). Inherited factors appear to be influential in extreme longevity, such as beyond 90 years for humans, even though this may at least in part be due to inheritance of healthy variants of genes instead of those predisposing to a specific disease, such as an apolipoprotein E gene allele, apoE4, shown to increase risk of cardiovascular and neurodegenerative diseases, or carcinogenic variants of BRCA1, a gene associated with breast cancer development.

DNA is the understandable focus of those exploring the nature of ageing and many current and previous theories address its biology. Of the vast number of chromosomal breakages which usually occur in cells, many are not repaired, and one theory proposes that ageing is primarily due to the effects of an accumulation of such damage to DNA (Medawar, 1952). Clearly the amount of redundancy in the genome of a species is relevant here. A theory of 'antagonistic pleiotropy' postulates that a few specific inherited genes, possibly with beneficial effects in the younger organism, exert multiple deleterious influences later in life (Williams, 1957). Central to some ageing theories is 'replicative senescence', a term describing the damaging outcomes resulting from the progressive loss of the protective chromosome ends (telomeres) (Joosten et al., 2003). Such telomere shortening usually occurs with each cell division and appears to be related to the finite number of divisions a cell can undergo. The fact that the enzyme telomerase causes elongation of telomeres, potentially reversing 'replicative senescence', has resulted in the telomerase-encoding gene being labelled one of the 'ageing genes'. Further interaction between genetic and stochastic factors and ageing and disease is indicated by influences such as radiation and interruption of blood supply increasing cell proliferation, arguably 'speeding up the clock', causing telomere shortening and thereby exposing the DNA to greater risk of randomly inflicted damage. Recent studies of fibroblasts indicate that ageing and associated disease may be slowed by removal of those cells which present a more senescent phenotype than others in the body, particularly as the cells secrete cytokines, which are potentially harmful to the structures around them (Burton, 2009). (*See below regarding cell ageing.)*

A 'disposable soma' theory proposes that finite energy and tissue is available to any organism and that this may be conserved or altered to some degree through different environmental conditions or genetic manipulations (Kirkwood, 1977).

Circadian rhythms change with age, resulting in less nocturnal lowering of temperature and metabolic rate (Hofman and Swaab, 2006; Chokroverty, 1999). A theory of 'upregulation failure' refers to research indicating that such loss of amplitude of temperature and metabolism cycles limits the ability of target cells to restore receptor functions after a normal diurnal decline following the usual exposure to various stimuli, and so contributes to the evident age change of diminished cell responses to certain neuroendocrine and cytokine controls (MacGibbon, 1996).

Other theories propose that ageing is a mainly a result of 'wear and tear' or autoimmune phenomena (Wilson et al., 2008).

Regimens shown to modulate ageing in various mammalian species have profoundly influenced ageing theory development. Some primary interventions include calorie restriction (CR) and neuroendocrine modification, such as replacement of certain hormones or reduction of others, including reproductive hormones, by removal of pituitary tissue or castration (Duffy et al., 1990; Everitt, 1973). The dramatic age-retarding effects of CR have elicited extensive research, including that of associated changes in mitochondrial function, hormonal levels and circadian rhythms, inflammation-related cytokines, rate of turnover of proteins such as enzymes and rate of stem cell depletion (Ungvari et al., 2008; Tavernarakis and Driscoll, 2002; MacGibbon, 2000; Weindruch, 1996). CR protocols generally require animals to eat approximately 65% of the usual caloric intake, resulting in lengthy fasting periods every day.

Some researchers propose that the restoration of youthful biorhythms and the potential associated benefits in relation to ageing and associated diseases may be achieved by interventions, including the adoption of fasting periods emulating those incurred by CR, or by exercise, hormone replacement or various other regimens. These theories are supported by numerous studies (Feuers et al., 1990). The pleiotropic nature of melatonin, which controls various hormone pathways and circadian rhythms, has resulted in much focus on this hormone in relation to ageing (Manda and Bhatia, 2004; MacGibbon et al., 2000). Although the underlying mechanisms may not be fully understood, the apparent benefits of exercise in retarding ageing and age-related conditions are well documented and much analysed, in particular the effects on the musculoskeletal and cardiovascular systems and on metabolic processes, including improvement in glucose homeostasis (Halverstadt et al., 2007; Ferrara et al., 2006; Joseph et al., 2005).

Human biological age changes

Where the following material reflects a general consensus in current primary gerontology and geriatric medical texts and peer-reviewed scientific publications it is not specifically referenced, while current texts which contributed to the development of this section are identified by asterisks in the reference list at the end of the book.

Overview of functional changes

This is where the rubber hits the road, so to speak, where ageing change is seen to affect performance. True age change appears to involve both a loss of rapid response to certain stressors and a decline in reserve.

Homeostatic responses are reduced, particularly in fight/flight situations and in infection and changes in blood sugar, hydration and temperature. These changes are associated with various structural and functional alterations, including an apparent sluggishness in the effector arms of the respective regulatory pathways, such as the target cell responses to catecholamines, insulin, glucagon, anti-diuretic hormone (ADH) and immune signals such as interleukin-2.

These alterations with age contribute to an increased susceptibility to hypoxia, dehydration, hyperglycemia, hyperthermia and hypothermia, respiratory and urinary infections and adverse effects of medication, as well as to a higher risk of surgical complications. They not only increase morbidity and mortality but, along with other factors, contribute to alteration in the presentation of disease.

Reduced reserve, such as in the respiratory and renal systems, makes an otherwise well older person much more likely than their younger counterpart to die as a result of infection or surgery, due to the associated increase in demands on their organ systems. A new intense challenge to an old body may be comparable to 'the straw that broke the camel's back' with one more stress causing the other organ systems to fail as their reserve capacity is exceeded.

Ageing is commonly associated with profound change in presentation of pathology and in pharmacokinetics and pharmacodynamics, in part related to normal age changes, including the altered responses and reduced reserve, and in part to disease processes.

As discussed above, greater variation occurs between individuals with increasing age, with some, for example, manifesting more youthful renal function than others. Also, within an individual, the rate of overall ageing may change, and may occur at a faster rate in certain systems and cells than others. Such diversity contributes significantly to the complexity of geriatric medicine, such as in diagnosis and in predicting a response to a drug. Two people of the same age and overt similarity in health status may markedly differ in hepatic and renal function with associated differences in metabolism and excretion of certain drugs. Some older individuals may also manifest pathology with the signs and symptoms more typical of a younger adult while, as mentioned, many others do not.

It is important to note that some age changes may suit the context of the older body. For example, a very youthful, relatively aggressive immune system may tend to delete too many older cells which are slightly altered, but which still serve a useful function and may be essential as cell numbers diminish. Also, with regard to modifying this change, certain interventions intended to boost defence responses have been found to be cancer promoting. However, the indications that some senescent cells may harm other cells, with many other problems potentially addressed by modified immune activities, make more selective restoration of this system worth further investigation.

Cell and tissue changes

Cell turnover is slower, potentially resulting in an increase in those cells with damaged molecules due to effects of free radicals and other agents. Longer cell cycles also contribute to a slower tissue repair. Structurally, many cell changes are found, and include an increase in nucleoli, reduced telomere length and increased incidence of aneuploidy. The pigment, lipofuscin, accumulates, especially in non-mitotic cells such as cardiac myocytes which, as a result, turn brown with age. However, this substance appears primarily to have a cluttering effect with minimal functional consequences. The more functionally significant cellular changes appear to be the alterations in both the cell membrane and postmembrane components of signalling pathways in the secretion of cytokines,[2] in mitochondrial respiratory chain function and in important molecules such as DNA, including the breakages and telomere changes discussed earlier.

Some of the age-related system changes clearly relate to alterations in histology and body composition. Significant changes include, as a percentage of total body mass:

- ↓ in muscle, often referred to as 'lean mass', and an associated
- ↓ in basal energy, consumption and water volume in the body;
- ↑ in fat, although this is not always obvious as fat increases in and around viscera and skeletal muscles, while hypodermal fat diminishes.

The effects of these changes include a loss of insulating fat in the skin and altered volumes of distribution for both drugs and endogenous molecules such as hormones.

---

2 Some current research indicates that in mitotic tissues certain 'senescent cells', described as having undergone an irreversible cell cycle arrest, accumulate and damage the healthier, growth-competent 'quiescent' cells and extracellular components surrounding them by the secretion of pro-inflammatory cytokines and upregulation of enzymes capable of degrading proteins (Burton, 2009).

In most tissues, cell numbers decline and parenchymal (functional) tissue is replaced by collagen and, in some areas, by adipose tissue. Collagen, the primary structural protein in the body, becomes predictably stiffer with an associated loss of compliance, such as in arteries, tendons and intercostal cartilages. Elastin loses elasticity and strength with various significant functional outcomes also in the cardiovascular, respiratory and other systems. The large arteries are less able to dilate as much during systole, although they are a little wider during diastole, with less elastic recoil, and these factors may contribute to the higher systolic pressure and an increase in cardiac workload found in normal ageing. In the respiratory system, the collagen changes are associated with diminished rib expansion and an associated dependence on diaphragmatic breathing. The earlier closing of bronchioles during exhalation and increased residual volume are thought to result largely from a loss of elastin properties of maintaining patency of small airways and enabling alveolar recoil. The elastin and collagen changes are primarily due to the formation of cross-linkages, such as disulphide bonds, between adjacent molecules. Various animal studies have found that collagen cross-linking and an associated loss of elasticity increases linearly with age (Everitt et al., 1980) and, due to collagen elasticity being relatively easy to measure, this variable has been considered to be 'one of the best biomarkers of the ageing process' (Holliday, 1995).

System changes

Apart from certain specific examples, such as the dramatic reproductive age change in females, most systems manage to perform their roles reasonably well in the ageing individual until late old age if not presented with extreme demands, but all are susceptible to malfunction when required to markedly intensify or adapt their functions.

Integumentary ageing

The skin, primarily due to dermal changes, becomes thinner, more transparent and less elastic. Epidermal cell replacement is slower. Adipose tissue in the hypodermis reduces, oil secretion declines and sweat glands reduce in number with those remaining being slower to activate. The production of both vitamin D and melanin is reduced. Perfusion of integumentary tissues declines and dermal blood vessels are less responsive to autonomic regulation. Actinic (sun) damage generally accelerates much of skin ageing (Jenkins, 2002).

The consequences of these age changes include a decrease in insulation properties and thermoregulation, a drier skin more prone to pruritis and infection, slower healing and reduced ability to contribute to altered hemodynamics in various physiological circumstances, such as those involving sympathetic stimulation. The skin becomes less reliable as an indicator of systemic dehydration. The colour changes with age are mainly due to reduction in perfusion and melanin production.

Hair becomes thinner, more brittle and loses its natural colour. An increase in facial hair occurs in women. Nails become thicker and often harder. Skin changes are thought also to contribute to reduced somasthetic sensory responses, including those to certain painful stimuli, although such changes appear to vary markedly between individuals.

Nervous system ageing

Cognitive functions with normal ageing are only subtly altered, although they are more susceptible to impairment, temporary or permanent, when unusual and pathological stresses are placed on the body. However, some autonomic functions clearly decline, as manifested in the poor adaptation to fight/flight requirements and sluggish adrenergic responses. Certain special and somasthetic sensory changes occur, and are discussed briefly below.

Various gross and histological changes are found in the brains of those who aged and died without apparent functional pathology, and the significance of these structural changes is not well established. Lipofuscin accumulates but, as in other tissues, without apparent functional significance. Some histological changes are found similar to those seen to a more extreme degree in brains of those who had Alzheimer's disease (AD). These include neurofibrillary tangles, plaques, some hippocampal degeneration and some synaptic alterations in the same circuits. However, all major research concludes that AD is not just exaggerated ageing. A general consensus is that all confusion and dementia are manifestations of specific pathology and are not part of normal ageing, even though, as indicated, the threshold for delirium in particular is much lower in the older individual due in part to reduced reserve (see below).

Although much variation in brain structural changes is observed in apparently normal individuals, common changes include a reduction in brain weight by approximately 20% by age 90, a decrease in neuron numbers (according to most studies) and a 15–20% reduction in the synapses in the frontal lobes.

A recent study of the frontal and temporal neocortical regions of brains of those who died without evidence of dementia found clear evidence of an age-related cortical thinning while total neuronal numbers in these regions remained constant, suggesting volume loss was due to change in neuronal and dendritic architecture (Freeman et al., 2008). A study of MRI scans of brains of 93 healthy people aged 18 to 93 found that white matter degraded with age, mainly in the connections between the anterior and posterior regions and, of the older cohort, disruptions in white matter integrity were correlated with some reduction in cognitive performance across a range of domains (Andrews-Hanna et al., 2007).

As in ageing of other systems, diversity in what are considered to be normal cognitive changes is generally found between individuals in the same age group, such as that indicated by the MRI study. The functional changes which are observed more clearly after approximately 75 years involve some decline in learning and memory ability, in intelligence as determined in IQ tests and in reaction time. However, while marked alteration in brain function, such as an inability to think clearly and serious memory loss, is not normal, some range in cognition occurs in the older generation, and in certain older adults any such decline must be extremely minimal.

Age changes seen in the histology of the hypothalamic suprachiasmatic nucleus (SCN), a critical component in determining circadian rhythms, are thought to be central to the observed disruption and loss of amplitude in the usual 24 hour cycles of hormonal rhythms, core temperature and sleep patterns seen in normal ageing (Hofman and Swaab, 2006). (*See ageing theories.*)

The sleep pattern changes result in shorter, lighter and more broken sleep periods, reducing the quality of sleep and predisposing the older individual to daytime sleepiness and, especially where other stresses are present also, to loss of concentration, impairments in decision making, memory problems and the 'Geriatric Giants' of confusion and falls. A tendency both to go to sleep and to wake earlier is observed. More time is spent in the lightest kind of sleep (stage 1) and much less in the deepest and most restorative kinds of sleep (stages 3 and 4), with some researchers stating that these stages are rarely achieved in older individuals. Some research indicates rapid eye movement sleep is reduced and some that it is unchanged and merely occurs earlier in the sleep cycle. Reported non-pharmacological interventions which encourage deeper sleep include regular daily routines, exercise and being exposed to normal outdoor light, particularly later in the day.

Alterations in reflexes, balance and gait, involving central and peripheral nervous, sensory and musculoskeletal systems, occur and aspects of these are discussed below. Reflexes are generally less brisk, especially in the lower extremities. A clinically-insignificant tremor commonly affects the upper extremities, head and voice.

Sensory ageing

Although the changes listed below are primarily considered to be sensory organ changes some may reflect alteration in central nervous system function.

Vision and the eyes

Presbyopia, an inability to focus on near objects, is considered to be a true age change and to result primarily from a loss of lens elasticity. Some yellowing of the lens also occurs, and is thought to reduce perception in blue light. This is also indicated in the painting colours used by ageing artists. Pupils tend to become smaller and accommodation is slower both to light and dark. Sensitivity to glare increases, for example, resulting from shiny floors or oncoming headlights. Bright, indirect lighting is recommended for activities such as reading. Arcus senilis is common but is not considered significant.

Hearing and the ears

Normal age change includes presbycusis, a loss of ability to hear high frequency sounds such as those of consonants b, t and d. Difficulty in hearing in the presence of background noise, a phenomenon described as 'recruitment', occurs, especially if the noise is loud. When talking to older people one should enunciate consonants clearly, as words without them sound meaningless. In some instances it is also a good idea to talk relatively slowly without speaking more loudly, while remembering that cognitive functions in interpreting speech are normally unaffected in any significant way. Ear wax becomes more viscous and dry, and sometimes needs to be cleared.

Taste and smell

Both diminish, with a general decrease occurring in ability to taste, with sour and bitter tastes declining the most, while elevated thresholds occur for smell detection and recognition. A challenge in menu preparation is to make food attractive and tasty without increasing salt or sugar with their respective causal links with hypertension and diabetes.

Vestibular and somasthetic senses

A reduction in vestibular sense and some decline in proprioception, in conjunction with other neural and musculoskeletal changes, result in impaired balance, predisposing the older individual to falling. Decline is observed in sensitivity to touch, two-point discrimination and high-frequency vibration. Pain perception findings are diverse, for example, some research reports a range of loss of integumentary pain while others find that it is usually intact. Considerable variation is also found in pain manifestations of disorders such as angina and infections, as discussed briefly later in this book.

Respiratory ageing

Respiratory function is normally maintained at rest, with tidal volume remaining much the same and a slight to no increase in resting respiratory rate. Age changes appear primarily to limit ability to markedly increase gas exchange and to counter respiratory infection. The afore-mentioned reduction in chest cage compliance and loss of the lung elastin functions of recoil and maintenance of patency of small airways contribute to a diminished total lung capacity, increase in air trapping and more diaphragmatic breathing. These, together with the extrapulmonary and autonomic changes addressed below, result in various other measurable changes in ventilation, including an increase in residual volume, decreases in forced vital capacity (FVC), forced expiratory volume in 1 second

(FEV1), peak expiratory flow rate and respiratory reserve. The elastin deterioration causes the lungs to be a little more compliant, slightly compensating for the more rigid thoracic cage. Other extrapulmonary changes limiting ventilation include reduction in intervertebral disc size, reduced strength and endurance in the muscles of ventilation and increased anterior-posterior diameter of the thorax. Dead space increases due to both a general increase in diameter of the airways and a reduction in alveolar surface area. This, with the premature closing of airways, contributes to a ventilation-perfusion mismatch. Airway defences are impaired, especially that of mucociliary function in the lower airways.

Collectively, these changes, together with the reduced adrenergic responses both in this system (affecting bronchodilation and other functions) and in other systems, contribute to the decline in ability of the older individual to respond to intense and sudden increased demand for oxygen. This also exacerbates the reduced lymphocyte-mediated response against infections such as flu and pneumonia. The decline in beta-adrenoceptor activity has also been postulated as aetiological in late-onset asthma (Connolly et al., 1995).

Cardiovascular ageing

Numbers of myocardial cells decline and those remaining hypertrophy, while lipofuscin and collagen accumulate within them. The protein amyloid is deposited extracellularly. Atrial pacemaker cells reduce in number and some fibrosis occurs in the conduction pathway. Also, some valve calcification occurs, affecting mainly the aortic valve, although this is commonly asymptomatic. The left ventricle becomes hypertrophic and its diastolic compliance is reduced. A decrease in response to beta-adrenergic stimulation occurs.

As stated above, the large arteries, including the aorta, widen and lengthen but are less compliant and have reduced elastic recoil. These factors would tend to contribute to the increase in afterload and the ventricular hypertrophy found to occur with age.

An increase in systolic pressure is generally associated with normal ageing, while diastolic pressure and resting heart rate usually remain the same. Although a systolic pressure increase is considered normal, the risk of pathology resulting from any hypertension is such that current medical protocols generally propose that 'high-normal' blood pressure (130-139/85-89) warrants life style modification even in the absence of any other symptoms. If any evidence of cardiovascular disease or target organ damage is also present, or if blood pressure is any higher, then antihypertensive medication is also recommended.

Age changes increase the work load of the heart but cardiac function at rest is not markedly altered. However, a distinct decline is observed both in the response to a sudden requirement for increased cardiac activity and in the maximum function possible.

Regular exercise appears to help to minimise these functional changes.

Postural hypotension, once thought to be a true age change, is now considered to be a sign of pathology.

Endocrine ageing

Particularly important changes include insulin resistance, which creates a mild diabetogenic effect, and a decrease in responses to adrenergic stimuli (especially where beta receptors are involved), to ADH and to hormones countering low blood glucose such as glucagon, as well as the catecholamines. The secretion of melatonin and thymus hormones declines. By 65 years of age most women have been menopausal for many years, and the associated sustained low oestrogen and progesterone levels (particularly oestrogen) increase susceptibility to clinically-significant changes in various organ systems as well as the reproductive system. These include loss of bone matrix increasing susceptibility to fractures and a change in serum lipids to profiles which predispose to atherosclerosis. In some men a marked decline in testosterone occurs while others show no change. Although variation is seen, in both sexes an increase in FSH and LH is frequently associated with low levels of the primary sex hormones.

Some individuals show one or a combination of the following changes, several of which limit ability to maintain fluid and electrolyte balance and normal hemodynamics:- growth hormone, renin and aldosterone, and atrial natriuretic peptide (Nicholl et al., 2008).

Studies indicate that while serum levels of other hormones may remain relatively unchanged, this does not necessarily reflect youthful rates of their secretion or metabolism, but that the rates of formation and breakdown may be slower. Alteration in circadian rhythms of secretion has been demonstrated to occur with regard to certain hormones, while volumes of distribution are changed in part due to altered body composition. There is indication that some of these changes are linked to altered patterns of sleep, immune decline and various other systemic features of ageing. Aspects of such influences are discussed elsewhere in this chapter.

Gastrointestinal ageing

Although some structural atrophy occurs and gastric acid secretion is reduced, the older gastrointestinal system shows little significant functional change with age, particularly if a healthy diet and exercise regimen are maintained. Caloric requirements generally decline due to a reduction in both exercise and lean body mass.

Teeth problems and poor dentistry can result in poor nutrition and were once a common feature of ageing associated with anaemia. However, in advanced societies this is not now considered a major cause of malnutrition.

Impaired swallowing, formerly thought to be a true age change and hence called presbyesophagus, is now thought to be associated with disease.

Hepatic function for normal requirements is also generally maintained, although those changes which do occur can be significant in metabolism of certain drugs (see below).

The significance of rigorous maintenance of a healthy diet is reinforced by the research discussed in the introduction regarding factors associated with longevity and ageing, and by clear evidence that high sugar intake is an independent risk factor for diabetes mellitus. The 'Australian Guide to Healthy Eating' on the Commonwealth Government Department of Health and Ageing website reflects major principles of good nutrition, including specific recommendations for those in the 65 years and older age groups (see references). Some major features listed are the selection of those complex carbohydrates with a low glycaemic index, limitation of simple sugars and salt and reduced caloric intake. Certain more common age-related conditions such as constipation and anaemia[3] reinforce the need for adequate intake of iron, vitamin B12 and insoluble fibre, together with exercise and adequate water intake. More details of recommended nutrition for healthy ageing are discussed elsewhere in this book.

---

3 Although sometimes associated with more serious pathology, anaemia is usually attributed to mild, clinically insignificant occult intestinal bleeding.

Renal ageing

Renal mass frequently declines, with more atrophy occurring in the cortical than the medullary regions. Glomeruli are lost, and of those remaining some become sclerosed. Renal perfusion lessens, more so in the cortex than the medulla.

A reduction in renal function is considered to be usual, although, as stated earlier, much variation is found, with some individuals retaining relatively youthful kidney status. Serum urea levels are usually reported to be unchanged. However, this is not considered to reflect particularly healthy nephrons but rather to be due to reduced protein metabolism resulting from a reduction in any or all of the following: muscle mass, protein intake and hepatic function. Similarly, due to reduced muscle bulk, low serum creatinine is not considered as reliable as the creatinine clearance rate in indicating degree of renal function. (*Note:* The serum level of Cytastin C, a protein produced by all cells and excreted in urine, is currently being reviewed as possibly a better indicator of renal status than serum creatinine.)

The older kidney typically develops isothuria, a condition in which urine concentration remains generally constant regardless of over- or under-hydration, the poor response to the latter partly explained by a diminished response to ADH. Nocturia is common, in part explained by the inability of the older kidney to process a large water load quickly, but also possibly due to a loss of diurnal rhythm in urine formation. Incontinence is predisposed by this and by various other age changes, including diminished bladder capacity and incomplete bladder emptying.

The usual loss of renal reserve can result in rapid renal failure when systemic or renal pathology places extreme demands on the kidney.

Musculoskeletal ageing

Although some ageing individuals remain fit and flexible enough to run marathons into their 70s, changes in these systems generally affect mobility and, together with reduced autonomic responses preclude sudden, intense activity such as sprinting.

Major changes include:

- ↓ number of muscle cells, resulting in ↓ lean body mass;
- diminished muscle strength;
- stiffer joints, associated with collagen changes

(Note: osteoarthritis, although common, is not inevitable and not considered to reflect a 'true' ageing change); and

- ↓ bone matrix, predisposing the individual to osteoporosis and fractures.

Bones weaken as resorption exceeds bone formation, causing a loss of matrix especially in trabecular bone while the remaining matrix appears normal in its composition. In long bones the shaft diameter increases but the medullary cavity widens, resulting in a net thinning of cortical bone.

Regular exercise can help to limit both bone and muscle atrophy but some loss of functional tissue is inevitable. In the remaining muscle tissue the fibres are less effective, with fat, collagen and lipofuscin deposition occurring. Gaining muscle mass with exercise does not incur as much increased muscle strength as it does in younger adults and mitochondrial changes cause some decline in aerobic respiration (Goodpaster, 2006).

The decline in muscle strength and nervous system changes together result in reduced reaction time and slower reflexes, including those of balance, posture and movement. Gait is less regular and efficient, involving a shorter stride and less arm swing, with women tending to develop a 'waddling', narrow-based gait with more body sway, and men a more wide-based gait. These factors predispose the older individual to falls.

Some small reduction in height is usual and is variously ascribed to reduced fluid in the intervertebral discs, loss of vertebral tissue, altered curvature of the spine and increased flexion of the knees and hips.

Reproductive ageing

Endocrine changes are discussed above, including the postmenopausal serum profile of reproductive hormones in women and the considerable diversity of these hormones in men. The latter is partly demonstrated by some nonagenarians fathering children. In males the prostate usually increases in size, sometimes impeding micturition. In women oestrogen decline is associated with atrophy of reproductive organs including thinning of the vagina wall as well as change in vaginal secretions, together resulting in a greater propensity for bleeding, dryness and thrush, as well as changes in other systems, particularly skeletal and haematological. Although sexual response decreases, healthy ageing does not necessarily result in cessation of sexual activity in either sex.

Immune ageing

Changes within each system contribute to the decline in resistance to disease, in particular to infection. Specific alterations in the immune system probably contribute to the increase in susceptibility to diseases such as flu and pneumonia, to some decrease in response to vaccination and to an apparent reactivation of some quiescent infections such as tuberculosis and chickenpox. Specific immune changes include a reduction in lymphoid tissue, smaller lymph nodes, thymic involution (although thymic remnants may remain active until extreme old age) and a decrease in both humoral and cell-mediated immunity, associated especially with a decline in response to the cytokine interleukin-2. Some decline in neutrophil and macrophage phagocytic ability is observed. Certain autoantibodies increase but their significance is unclear.

The blood and ageing

Peripheral blood films are usually relatively unchanged and specific structural changes observed in erythrocytes and most leukocytes are not considered to be very significant functionally. However, as stated above, lymphocyte response to stimuli is reduced and some phagocytic function of other leukocytes declines. Research findings are conflicting, but plasma proteins are generally thought to be maintained overall, with low levels considered to reflect pathological change. Haemopoietic tissue declines, but that which remains is found to be normal in composition and in response to stimuli such as erythropoietin. Lipid profiles are seen to change, particularly in women, in association with a reduction in sex hormones.

Age changes which affect pharmacokinetics and pharmacodynamics

It is important to remember that considerable differences occur between older individuals during apparently normal ageing, with some manifesting youthful function in certain variables, including creatinine clearance. Some individual differences in response to drugs may, of course, reflect aspects of specific pathology.

A commonly used estimate of creatinine clearance for men is:

_(140 - age)xlean body weight (kg)/72x serum creatinine (x0.85 for women)

However, actual creatinine clearance assessment is much more reliable.

The BLSA found a correlation between a decline in glomerular filtration rate (GFR) and hypertension. It also found that, in the absence of diseases known to impair function, GFR remained stable in 1/3 of older adults over a 24-year period.

Change with age in kinetics and receptor response occurs with many drugs. The following are commonly observed features, with examples of commonly-used drugs listed below:

- ↓ absorption rate, particularly if the drug depends on low pH (e.g. calcium);
- ↓ lean mass and body water and ↑ adipose tissue as a percentage of body mass. These are especially significant regarding the volume of distribution (VD) for water soluble drugs with the risk of higher concentrations (e.g. digoxin and thiazide) and the longer retention and half-life of fat-soluble drugs with associated risks (e.g. diazepam);
- A possible ↓ in plasma albumin, increasing the free (active) form of those drugs which normally bind to this protein (e.g. phenytoin, digoxin, aspirin and warfarin). This change is especially observed in unhealthy older individuals;
- An age-related inefficiency in the blood-brain barrier is described in some texts, with this change possibly enabling drugs to enter the brain more

easily, warranting more careful monitoring of patients when administering psychoactive drugs in particular;

- ↓ hepatic clearance due to both ↓ perfusion and altered metabolism. Phase 1 hepatic metabolism functions of oxidation, reduction and hydrolysis appear to be more impaired with age than the phase 2 conjugative/synthetic reactions. Ageing also affects certain isoforms of cytochrome P450 influencing drugs such as diazepam, piroxicam, theophylline and quinidine. The decreased perfusion is considered to especially reduce the metabolism of drugs which are subjected to a high first-pass effect, including imipramine, lidocaine and propranolol;
- ↓ renal clearance usually affecting digoxin, angiotensin-converting enzyme (ACE) inhibitors, acetazolamide, amantadine, aminoglycosides, furosemide, metformin, ranitidine, vancomycin and morphine sulphate;
- ↓ target cell response to certain drugs including beta-adrenoceptors, furosemide and vaccines; and
- ↑ target cell response to certain drugs including warfarin, anticholinergics, H1 blockers and psychoactive drugs (e.g. benzodiazepines, neuroleptics and opioids). Note: calcium channel blockers cause ↑ response in control of blood pressure but ↓ response in atrioventricular blockage. (This may be due to differing age changes in the alpha-compared with beta-adrenoceptors.)

The hazards of polypharmacy, as discussed in later chapters, can be exacerbated by many of these age-related changes (e.g. where drugs compete for serum protein-binding when the primary serum protein, albumin, may be reduced).

Age changes relating to altered presentations in pathology

As stated above, any new stress in an old body, such as dehydration, may be 'the final straw', with one intense demand pushing the organs beyond their reserve capacity. As one system fails, its effects can create a chain reaction as greater loads are placed on the others.

You will be learning in later chapters about the Geriatric Giants of confusion, falling, incontinence and immobility as common presentations. Any sudden appearance of one of these, if not accompanied by a cardiac arrest or stroke or any sudden psychological stress or new medication, is most likely to be due to an infection. The muted and sometimes contradictory manifestations of conditions in the older patient may be related to some age changes.

Primary among these are thought to be combinations of the following changes, most of which have been discussed above:

- ↓ autonomic beta-adrenoceptor response causing, for example, less ↑ HR in stress response;

- ↓ reserve (e.g. in respiratory and renal systems) so that any added need, such as sudden ↑ in oxygen requirement may not be met predisposing to hypoxia, confusion, cardiac problems etc. (Usually, for every 10C ↑ in temperature oxygen needs to by approximately 13%.);
- The loss of reserve includes loss of cells with deterioration frequently observed in those remaining;
- ↓ volume regulation – due to:
    - ↓ body water as % of body weight and therefore ↓ body reserves of water;
    - ↓ thirst drive (more likely to be a manifestation of specific pathology rather than ageing);
    - ↓ ADH response; and
    - ↓ renal function;

These lead to earlier and faster dehydration due to age and associated electrolyte problems, adding to confusion and other complications;

- ↓ blood sugar regulation;
- ↓ immune function (this may contribute to ↓ in classic symptoms of infection); and
- ↓ thermoregulation and possibly ↓ basal body temperature.[4]

---

4 Some studies indicate that older individuals may be cooler, with a basal temperature of up to approximately 10C less than that of younger individuals. The conclusions made are that protocols for assessment of fever or hyperthermia in the older should be changed accordingly. Proposed causes for temperature decline

A final comment

Age-modulating regimens involving telomerase, senescent cell apoptosis, stem cell replacement or other interventions could one day become common and change ageing as we know it. In the meantime some mode of ageing is inescapable, whether primarily due to 'true ageing' or to disease.

Older adults, often formidable and strong in many respects, are nonetheless more vulnerable due to those age changes which can make them become seriously ill and can result in death when an infection strikes or a stressor is sudden and intense. Extreme and abrupt changes in tissue oxygen needs, temperature, hydration or blood sugars should be avoided where possible. Such changes are inherent in sudden exertion, where the reduced autonomic response and other features of ageing increase the chances of hypoxia of vital organs and myocardial infarction. Dehydration, a common occurrence in older individuals, can have devastating effects, with an associated electrolyte imbalance,

---

include decrease in muscle activity, meal-induced brown fat metabolism and thyroid hormone action. (See UNMC weblink references.) However, more recent research indicates that a clear correlation between ageing and lowered basal temperature is not established, and that more research is needed to also address gender, ambient temperature and the body site where temperature is measured (Lu and Dai, 2008; Sund-Levander et al., 2002).

stress on the ageing kidneys and the potential for increased viscosity and clotting of the blood.

However, for the normally-ageing individual, focussing on the difficulties of ageing may be counterproductive, as, to age successfully, the primary advice from many gerontological authorities is not only to have a good diet and regular medical check-ups but to explore new challenges and exercise robustly. Possibly one's 'philosophy of life' will determine how this issue is approached.

No discussion about normal biological ageing in humans would be complete without acknowledgement of the considerable impact of psychosocial factors. Some researchers consider these to be better predictors than physical variables of how well an individual will age biologically. It is of course important not to confuse correlation and causality. The finding that bingo players have reduced AD, or the BLSA results of the super-centenarians study in which all cognitive domains tested were associated with frequency of engagement in non-physical hobbies (Willcox et al., 2008), may not demonstrate causal relationships. However, where strong correlations between psychosocial and behavioural factors and markers of healthy ageing are found they should not be ignored. Positive feedback cycles may be postulated, linking variables such as motivation, exercise, appetite, social interaction, music and academic pursuits, with causal pathways involving such factors as endorphins, enhanced glucose homeostasis and restoration of youthful biorhythms. The corollary also applies, where isolation or poor nutrition may create cycles involving depression or impaired health.

As a final example, here is someone who possibly enjoys expression of fine genes, but also exhibits many of the postulated predictors of successful ageing which can be adopted by most of us, such as exercise and a healthy weight and attitude, including some denial of ageing:

Dot, the wonderful and very fit 80 year-old who climbed the Three Sisters cliff face in the Australian Blue Mountains, said at the time, 'I never considered myself old. I was young until I was thirty, and then I was an adult' (ABCTV, 1991).

Useful resources

Major journals include the *Journal of Gerontology,* and *Mechanisms of Ageing and Development.* Primary texts include the *Handbook of Biology of Ageing* series and other texts listed below and indicated with an asterisk, as well as Brocklehurst's *Textbook of Geriatric Medicine and Gerontology,* 7th edition, due for release in 2010.

Several useful websites:

Telomeres and ageing, and other ageing concepts – (this link, although sophisticated and new, may contain some erroneous material): http://www.whyweage.com/node/11

Normal brain ageing: http://www.med.harvard.edu/AANLIB/cases/caseA/case.html (to be viewed in conjunction with http://www.sbirc.ed.ac.uk/documents/ageing-brain-paper.pdf)

The Australian Government website on nutrition – refer to the PDF of the booklet – http://www.health.gov.au/internet/main/publishing.nsf/Content/health-pubhlth-publicat-document-fdcons-cnt.htm

'Geriatric Nursing' issues including normal ageing: http://consultgerirn.org

Relating age changes to altered presentation of pathology (from the University of Nebraska Medical Centre): http://webmedia.unmc.edu/intmed/geriatrics/pdf/ev_atypic.pdf

Gerontology Video Lectures – audiovisual quality is not good but content is: NIH 2001. http://bio-alive.com/seminars/gerontology.htm

Video:

Regarding 'Dot' as well as other normal ageing and clinical geriatric issues: *The Time of Your Life* by David Goldie, Oasis films, 1991, shown on ABCTV

Chapter 5

Health assessment of the older adult in Aotearoa New Zealand

Professor Rose McEldowney
Head of School of Health Sciences, CDU;
previously Associate Professor in Nursing,
Director of the Cultural Safety Research Unit,
Graduate School of Nursing and Midwifery,
Victoria University of Wellington, New Zealand

Objectives:

This chapter will enable the reader to:

1) identify the importance of cultural safety and appropriateness of health care provision for older adults;
2) demonstrate an understanding that older adults should participate to their fullest in decisions about their health and wellbeing;
3) examine the socio-economic inequalities that impact on the health and wellness of older adults; and

4) discuss assessment tools that have been developed for older adults and identify their assessment domains and dimensions.

Introduction

The World Health Organisation (2007) suggests that the worldwide growth in the numbers of older adults can be seen as a sign of improving global health influencing longevity. Although Aotearoa[5] New Zealand has a relatively young population compared to other OECD countries, the number of older people is increasing steadily. The estimated 2009 numbers of adults aged 65 years and over (based on prediction from the 2006 census) numbers 538,049 or 12.8% of the total population. By 2031 it is expected to have reached 22%.

In New Zealand older age is defined as adults 65 years of age and over. This is linked to the age at which New Zealanders are currently eligible for National Superannuation. However, Mãori (the Indigenous people of Aotearoa), Pacific Nations people and those with pre-existing disabilities are defined as being older adults at 55 years and over because of their life expectancy is shorter than that of other population groups (Ministry of Health (MoH), 2006). Pacific Nations people include those who were born to Pacific

5 Aotearoa is the Maori translation for New Zealand: 'Land of the long white cloud'.

families in New Zealand or those who migrated from the main island groups of Samoa, Tonga, Tokelau, the Cook Islands, Niue, Tuvalu and Fiji. Other, smaller ethnic groups include people from Kiribati, the Solomon Islands, Papua New Guinea and American Samoa. Over the next 50 years it is expected that Maori and Pacific older people aged 65 and over will also have increased proportionally by 270% and 400% respectively (MoH, 2006), although at this time the proportion of older Pacific people who are New Zealand born is small. Therefore one of the key considerations in the provision of health care for the older adult is that services need to be culturally safe and appropriate to meet the needs of an increasingly diverse older population.

The Ministry of Health is the major governmental health planning and funding agency in New Zealand. In the document Health of Older People Strategy (2006), which is informed by the *New Zealand Public Health and Disability Act 2000,* a vision for health care and diverse service delivery to promote positive ageing by 2010 is proposed; 'Older people participate to their fullest ability in decisions about their health and wellbeing and in family, whanau[6] and community life. They are supported in this by coordinated and responsive health and disability support programmes.' (p.1)

---

6 Whanau is the Maori translation of family, extended family.

To achieve this vision guiding principles are identified that relate to the following: informed choice; quality and integration of programmes to meet needs; timely access to funding and service delivery (including primary and community services); culturally appropriate services; promotion of health and wellbeing in the older population; seamless continuum of primary, secondary and tertiary care systems between home/community/hospital; and access to flexible coordinated support for family, whanau and carers (2006, pp.1-3). This strategy has also been informed by other key health documents and population and service based strategies such as Primary Health Care, Palliative Care, Mental Health, Maori Health – He Korowai Oranga and Pacific Health (MoH, 1998; MoH, 2001a, 2001b, 2001c; MoH, 2002).

Where does health care of the older adult take place? Most older people live healthy and active lives either in their own homes, in retirement villages and supported communities or with extended family or whanau. A minority of older adults who are frail and vulnerable require ongoing care and support due to chronic illness or disability. Socio-economic inequalities over time – for example, low-income, economic stress, high accommodation costs, poor housing, low status occupation and being Maori or Pacific – impact living standards and are key determinants of poor health in older age (Fergusson et al., 2001). The services required to support the person and whanau/family/carers within the home/community/hospital continuum may include supported accommodation, injury prevention, specialist medical and psychiatric care, palliative care, hospital care, assessment and rehabilitation, community support, equipment, respite and residential care. Nurses working in the community and aged care settings are in an ideal situation to assess the needs of older people and their whanau/family and plan for appropriate, accessible and affordable interventions and support. So how are the health care needs of older adults assessed, and what assessment frameworks are available to guide us? In this chapter an assessment framework is provided to assess the health needs of the older person. A practice story and guiding questions are also provided to support the learning process of assessing the older adult.

Assessment frameworks and tools

Assessment of the older adult includes several domains that have been identified in a systematic review of the literature (Martin and Martin, 2003). In Aotearoa New Zealand there are two frameworks or tools that have been implemented within residential, community and hospital settings - the computerised Inter Resident Assessment Instrument Mini Data Set-Home Care (InterRAI MDS-HC) assessment tool, and the Assessment of Older People with Complex Needs Framework developed by the New Zealand Guidelines Group and in their document Assessment Processes for Older People (2003) (www.nzgg.org.nz). The InterRAI MDS-HC was developed by a global network of over 40 researchers and clinicians from the InterRAI Organisation and recommended for implementation in New Zealand by the NZGG (NZGG, 2003). A comparison of the InterRAI MDS-HC against others assessment tools like the Mini Mental assessment tool (a geriatric assessment tool) concluded that the chosen tool was more complete in the assessment domains and content covered (NZGG, 2003). It is also one of the internationally validated and reliable tools used by District Health Boards (DHBs) to assess the health care needs of consumer groups (Hirdes, Ljunggren et al., 2008). Built upon the concept of a comprehensive standardised geriatric assessment the tool has been shown to improve health outcomes for older people in a variety of settings, especially when combined with long term management. The HC system is currently being used in North America, Europe, Asia, Australia and New Zealand (Heidenbohm et al., 2007).

The InterRAI MDS-HC tool consists of assessment and care planning processes that cover a multitude of domains for assessing older people, such as functional ability, mental/cognitive ability and social/environmental as well as the person's status in terms of cognition, communication, activities of daily living (ADL), continence, psychosocial well being, disease diagnosis and health conditions (Brant, Fries, Charles and Fahey, 2003; http://www.interrai.org/section/view/?fnode=15). Data collected from this assessment tool is integrated and appropriate information supports the continuum of care and promotes a link among carers who work in home and community areas, long-term care and acute and mental health care. The consistency of information enables health professionals and planners to promote and integrate services in a multidisciplinary and cost effective way.

Implementing the InterRAI MDS-HC tool and NZGG Assessment of Older People with Complex Needs Framework in practice

The assessment provides clinical information to patients and caregivers at the point of care, enabling a responsive approach to patient care. It consists of the MDS-HC and Clinical Assessment Protocols (CAPs). Items identified by the MDS-HC are called triggers that link to the CAPs which are general guidelines for how to respond to clients who may require further specialised assessment and individual care planning for a particular issue. For example, if a client at home is showing functional decline such as restricted mobility then a referral to an assessment and rehabilitation unit may be required to identify what might be contributing to the client's increasing frailty. Thomas (2001) and Fonda, Clipp and Maddox (2000) assert that functional status is highly valued by older people and closely associated with present and consequent health status. As the assessor the nurse needs to be aware of all the CAPs in order to plan care and refer to allied service providers as appropriate. A comprehensive assessment and recognition of the strengths and issues of the client can be useful as the nurse assessor schedules the treatment, care services and the care plan outcomes (InterRAI-HC, 2000).

The NZGG framework provides a comprehensive and complementary process to use alongside the MDS-HC database because it clearly identifies evidence-based domains and dimensions that need to be included by the nurse assessor and that can be identified at an early stage. According to the NZGG (2003) the areas of need that are most important for older people are personal care, social participation, control over daily life, food and safety. The domains and dimensions include:

1) **Physical health and functioning,** e.g. chronic illness; continence; nutrition; gait; mobility; cardiac, gastrointestinal, pulmonary, and cerebrovascular conditions; co-morbidities (diabetes); ADLs and IADLs including self-care and domestic abilities; iatrogenic disease (due to polypharmacy); sexual functioning; speech and language impairment; dental/oral health; vision and hearing.
2) **Mental health and functioning,** e.g. anxiety; depression and other mental illness; cognitive functioning; dementia; substance abuse; iatrogenic disease; emotional wellbeing.
3) **Social functioning,** e.g. financial status and management; housing; family/whanau support

and contact; social networks; social activities and supports.

4) **Presence and roles of carers.**
5) **Risk factors,** e.g. those aged 75 years and over; socially isolated/living alone; divorced/separated, never married, single or widowed; recently bereaved; no children; poor or limited economic resources; recent discharge from hospital; presenting at ED; recent change in health status; multiple disorders or illness; cognitively impaired; depression; poor health perception; high/low body mass index; lower extreme of functional impairment; low physical activity; taking 3 or more medications; sight/hearing impairment; elder abuse; alcohol/tobacco and/or substance abuse; carer under stress/change of carer/carer requests assessment of the older person.

However, while the InterRAI MDS-HC is purported to assess clients from an holistic perspective, there is an absence of focus on the cultural and ethnic diversity perspective. The NZGG acknowledges that in order to work in partnership with the older person with complex needs and their family or whanau, assessors need to be mindful about who should be assessed (refer to risk factors mentioned above) and how and where they should be assessed (e.g. older person including family/whanau and carers). For example, the group identifies the need to assess those aged 65 and over and Maori and Pacific people aged 55 and over. It is also recommended that when a

Maori older person chooses to be assessed using te reo Maori me ona tikanga (Maori language and protocols), a respected person fluent in the language is the most appropriate and safe assessor. The same is recommended for Pacific Nations clients.

In the next section a practice story about May – an 85 year old woman – is presented. Pseudonyms are used to protect the identity of the older person and her family.

A practice story

One afternoon, May arrives in the emergency department (ED) with a suspected fractured neck of femur. She has been at a family picnic down by the lake and was trying to catch a ball in a friendly game of cricket when she fell on hard ground. Her son Tom and daughter in law Louise (a nurse) support her to sit for a while and see if she can weight bear on her left leg. On rising from the chair May cannot stand properly so Louise decides to take her to the local hospital for assessment.

May lives in her small three bedroom home. She has been widowed for the past 25 years but has a strong local and extended family support network, as well as external social networks in the church and various women's clubs. She is also attached to her cat Poppy. May recently had to give up driving her car because she was unable to pass the sight test when her license was up for renewal. Her general practitioner is close by and she has been treated for right sided heart failure for about 10 years. Her medications consist of a diuretic, beta blocker and multivitamins.

On admission to ED, May is assessed by the orthopaedic registrar and an X-ray indicates she has a fractured neck of femur (NOF). She is admitted to the orthopaedic ward and goes to the OT (Operating Theatre) for insertion of a titanium head of femur.

On return to the ward May is doing well – her physiological assessment is within normal limits. Her nurse and physiotherapist mobilise her postoperatively on the second day. May is also very interested in her surroundings and likes to engage in conversation with other women in the 4 bed cubicle and with the nurses and other staff. Her family visit each day and respond to her requests for the newspaper, clothes and fruit. Unfortunately, during her time in hospital May's cat Poppy has gone missing and no-one has been able to locate her.

Five days into recovery the doctor and physiotherapist suggest that May go the rehabilitation unit which is 35 kilometres out of town. May becomes very distressed – she refuses to go and says, 'I really like it here so I've decided to stay – I'm not going home'. When Janet the social worker arrives to discuss the move with May and her daughter in law Louise, May becomes even more agitated and begins to lash out at Janet, saying, 'If you make me go I'll kill myself '. Louise is unable to ease the situation.

As the nurse looking after May, you undertake a nursing assessment using both the InterRAI-MD-SC tool and NZGG Assessment Framework. You check the patient notes and note that May has not been sleeping well during the night. She has been found wandering in and out of other patients' rooms. She has also been incontinent at times during the day and not interested in having a shower. You invite Louise and Tom to be present so the assessment is as comprehensive at it can be.

During the assessment you hear from Tom and Louise that May has recently required extra support in the home. When they call to see her she is often hungry and her house needs cleaning. They also notice that she is not going out very often.

For reflection

What are some of the key aspects that you will need to consider when assessing May's situation? Refer to the Domains of Assessment outlined in the New Zealand Guideline Group Assessment Framework (2003) and InterRAI MD-SC assessment tool. These can be downloaded on www.nzgg.org.nz and http://www.interrai.org/section/view/?fnode=15.

1) What is happening in May's situation that might cause her to behave differently?
2) How might you work with May and her family to identify what she needs?
3) What services may be useful to support May to transition from hospital to home?

Conclusion

Ageing is a dynamic process that is part of one's life course, but for some older adults it can present challenges to health and well-being. Being able to assess the needs of older adults is an essential aspect of nursing practice. The two validated assessment tools presented in this chapter provide a standardised approach to assessing the health needs of older adults within a hospital/community/home continuum.

However, caution is required when applying assessment tools and frameworks. While they are transferable between countries and health care systems, the key focus is that they be contextualised to suit individual older people and their circumstances. This also includes ensuring that the nurse assessor meets the cultural and ethnic components in a safe and competent way during the assessment and implementation stages.

Chapter 6

Evidence-based nursing practice

Professor Lynn Chenoweth
Professor of Aged and Extended Care, UTS, and Director, Health and Ageing Research Unit, South Eastern Sydney-Illawarra Area Health Service

Objectives:

This chapter will enable the reader to:

1) Demonstrate why decision-making and practice issues must be based on research evidence;
2) Discuss why a research culture in nursing is necessary;
3) Examine some of the reasons why nurses do not embrace evidence-based practice;
4) Evaluate the resources that are available to nurses to review evidence-based nursing practices;
5) Identify the major institutes for supporting evidence-based practice; and
6) Provide examples of evidence-based practice in aged care.

Introduction

In the current economic climate health and aged care services are required to demonstrate effectiveness and efficiency across all divisions, mandated by government-initiated policies and procedures that focus on monitoring the delivery of quality services. An important Australian Government policy involves implementing evidence-based health and aged care (Courtney, Rickard, Vickerstaff and Court, 2005, pp.3-7). Consequently, with dynamic policy changes occurring across health and aged care systems, health professionals are obliged to fully embrace evidence-based practice. It is no longer acceptable to rely exclusively on prior knowledge and experiences when making decisions about treatment and care. The concept of clinical governance explicitly requires that evidence-based practice is in day-to-day use to meet the health needs of patients/clients in the most efficient and effective way possible (National Health and Medical Research Council (NHMRC), 2000).

Context of evidence-based nursing practice

Many of the major structural and managerial changes recently introduced in the Australian health care system affect nursing practice, requiring nurses to take a more active role in ensuring effective patient/client outcomes. These changes have come about with the increasing longevity of the population, patient throughput and turnover, public awareness, access to health information and consumer expectations and the expansion of highly technical and expensive therapeutic approaches in health care treatments (McCormack, 2009). Since nurses are confronted every day with practice issues and the need to make sound decisions about patient/client care in this dynamic climate, there is a vital need to draw on research evidence in decision-making. Research provides the basis for making wise decisions about resource allocation, nursing interventions, patient/client assessments, understanding the effects of illness and disability and monitoring the patient's/client's reactions to these (Courtney, Rickard, Vickerstaff and Court, 2005, pp.5-7). Wise decision-making relies on gathering, analysing and synthesising the best evidence available on the topic of interest. Thus, the goal of evidence-based nursing is to enable nurses to carefully consider their care practices in light of the best available evidence for best-practice. Engaging in this process encourages nurses to systematically inquire into routine nursing practice and critically reflect on decisions made and actions taken. Indeed, the continuous development of nursing practice relies on nurses' willingness to employ these reflexive practices (Newman, Thompson and Roberts, 2006).

The international movement in evidence-based nursing has gained increasing momentum since the mid-1990s, with debate continuing on the relative merits of this approach in progressing professional nursing practice. Among the champions for evidence-based practice there is an unshakable belief in the capacity of science and the rational and systematic application of science to bring about effective, efficient and accountable health care practice. Champions posit that any difficulties associated with implementing evidence-based practice can be overcome by employing recommended approaches identified in systematic reviews of research evidence (Trinder, 2000, p 215). In contrast, the critics accuse evidence-based practice of being an overly simplistic and reductionist approach which fails to do justice to the inherent complexity of practice situations and thus may mislead the search for certainty (see, for example, Lancet, 1995).

In 1997 the Royal College of Nursing Australia (RCNA), spearheaded by Alan Pearson and colleagues at the University of Adelaide, put forward a discussion paper for consideration by the nursing profession outlining the philosophical base and the relative merits of implementing evidence-based health care practice. The authors commented that the main benefits to nursing and health consumers arising from evidence-based nursing is the opportunity to establish nursing interventions against best-practice guidelines in order to enable effective health outcomes measured against best-practice standards, and to practice nursing in a consistent way. In arguing for support of evidence-based practice, the RCNA (1997) reported the occurrence of a wide range of nursing interventions for preventing and treating pressure ulcers in 20 northern NSW hospitals, many of which were not based on the best available evidence. In part, this finding reflected nurses' tendency to rely on trial and error approaches in care and also to follow medical orders without question, rather than drawing on the evidence for recommending and employing optimal pressure ulcer treatments. This example highlighted nurses' unfamiliarity and uncertainty with the concept of evidence-based practice at the time.

Nevertheless, the need for a research culture in nursing had been recognised for many years, in particular a need for research questions to emerge from within the clinical context of nursing, rather than be imposed and investigated from without (Courtney, Rickard, Vickerstaff and Court, 2005). While recent government policy has mandated that evidence-based practice should occur mainly to create a more equitable, effective and efficient health system (Aged and Community Services Australia, 2007), the thrust of the argument for employing evidence-based nursing is about the development of professional practice leading to better health outcomes. First, research evidence enables nurses to describe and define their practice, and to identify the value that nursing care adds to patient/client outcomes. Second, evidence helps nurses to understand the influence and predict health outcomes as a result of nursing interventions. Both sets of evidence help nurses to take hold of and to be accountable for their practice (Burns and Grove, 2007).

Dimensions of evidence-based practice

The promotion of evidence-based practice for all health professionals stems from Cochrane's (1979) views in relation to evidence-based medicine, drawing his medical colleague's attention to the lack of information available on the effects of health care interventions. Cochrane's call to provide evidence of effectiveness was taken up by Sackett and colleagues (1995) from the University of Oxford in the mid 1990s. The subsequent development of evidence-based health care, developed initially in medicine, was based on three principles (National Institute for Clinical Excellence (NICE), 1996):

1) Health care staff must be taught how to interpret and use research findings;
2) Health care staff must be helped to use research to inform practice throughout their careers; and
3) Research findings must be disseminated to health care staff in more efficient ways.

(Website reference: www.nice.org.uk/article.asp?a=6834)

The urge to promote evidence-based medicine saw the emergence of the Cochrane Collaboration with the express aim of advancing evidence-based health care. This international network of individuals prepares, maintains and disseminates systematic and recent reviews of health care effects from a range of health interventions. The collaboration produces the Cochrane Library, a well-known database of systematic reviews of research, housing the Cochrane Database of Systematic Reviews (CDSR), available to the public free of charge on their website www.cochrane.org.

Many well-conducted reviews on drugs and other treatments generally prescribed for older people can be obtained from this website and provide valuable evidence upon which to make clinical decisions. For example, a Cochrane Collaboration review (2006) of placebo-controlled trials of the Alzheimer's disease drugs respiridone and olanzapine revealed a likelihood that aggression in dementia will decrease in the cases in which these drugs were used, compared to the placebo cases, and that respiridone may improve psychosis. The review findings are important since a previous study on these two drugs conducted by the National Institute of Mental Health (NIMH) (2001) identified that they afforded no benefit to people with Alzheimer's disease, with a subsequent reluctance of doctors to prescribe these treatments. The Cochrane review (2006), therefore, provided health consumers and their doctors with good evidence for making the important decision to invest in these treatments where suitable. Also, the publications obtained through the Cochrane Collaboration often contain valuable information that provides the necessary scientific evidence to help direct health policy decisions.

Another evidence-based support network, the NHS Centre for Reviews and Dissemination (CRD) in York, UK, provides services to promote awareness and access to quality research evidence reviews (www.york.ac.uk/inst/crd/welcome.htm) The National Institute for Clinical Excellence (NICE) works with clinical bodies to appraise health interventions and produce advice and guidelines for practice in specialist areas, such as nursing care of the older person (www.nice.org.uk).

Encouraging nurses to engage in evidence-based practice

There are many reasons why some nurses do not embrace evidence-based practice, although most nurses view research findings as 'legitimate' evidence, as opposed to evidence arising from direct clinical experiences (Rycroft-Malone, Harvey, Seers, Kitson, McCormack and Tichen, 2004). For nurses to embrace research arising from evidence-based practice they need to develop the skills to evaluate research, employ critical appraisal skills, keep up-to-date with research findings and disseminate research findings effectively to nursing colleagues. Lack of experience in conducting research inevitably deprives many nurses of the background knowledge and insight which could help them to make judgements about the validity, applicability and usefulness of the information produced by professional nursing and health publications (Rycroft-Malone, Harvey, Seers, Kitson, McCormack and Tichen, 2004). While newly-graduated nurses would have learnt about research methods and been encouraged to apply evidence during their practical experience programs, when entering the paid workforce and confronted by the realities of heavy caseloads and administrative demands these nurses say they have little time to engage in evidence-based nursing (Courtney, Rickard, Vickerstaff and Court, 2005, pp.16-19). Another reason is the problem with interpreting and using research products, with this often being viewed as too scientific and obscure, therefore lacking clinical credibility (McGaughan, Thompson, Callum, Sheldon and Thompson, 2002). Lack of organisational support to employ research findings is also a real issue for the busy clinician. However, having a multidisciplinary focus is a way of increasing the chances of research implementation in practice (Rycroft-Malone, Harvey, Seers, Kitson, McCormack and Tichen, 2004).

The factors identified can potentially stifle nurses' attempts to embrace evidence-based practice. However, nurses can draw on their familiarity with continuous quality improvement and clinical audit to gain the skills required to critically review their practice. Evidence-based nursing consists of five explicit steps:

1) The nurse, in caring for an individual patient/client, identifies a specific question about

their care. This could relate to a diagnosed problem, need or issue, the likely outcome of the problem, need or issue, the most effective nursing process required and the possible outcomes for the patient/client, resource use and so forth;
2) Finding the best evidence to answer these questions;
3) Evaluating the best evidence available for its usefulness and validity for the circumstances and the patient/client;
4) Applying the best nursing care identified for the patient/client to address the problem, need or issue; and
5) Evaluating and documenting the outcome of the nursing care implemented for the patient/client.

(Sackett, 1996; Kitson, Harvey and McCormack, 1998)

In any research endeavour the first step is to identify the clinical questions needed to proceed to a solution. Clinical questions focus on the patient/client characteristics, the actions that might need to be taken and the identification of a clear outcome or outcomes against which the action can be evaluated. Having identified these questions the next step is to find the best evidence relating to each question. This is often an overwhelming task for nurses due to the growing number of studies reported in nursing and health research journals that appear to be contradictory, or that are targeted to very specific aspects of care. Once relevant literature is obtained, these studies need to be critically appraised to evaluate the strength of the evidence reported. Validity is a term used to establish rigour in reported research, meaning the extent to which the results of the research are likely to be free from bias (Chang, 2009, pp.115-129). Specific methodological criteria have been identified for the evaluation of different types of research, and this is discussed later in this chapter. Once the quality and applicability of the research has been found suitable for implementation with a particular patient/client, the fourth step is to apply the research findings to their care and management, taking into account the patient's/client's own values and preferences. Evaluating the effects of this care and management is central to evidence-based nursing (Mott, Nolan, Zarb et al., 2004). Nurses are encouraged to continuously evaluate their own performance in relation to their use of evidence-based care and to ask whether the new care and management regimen is improving outcomes for the patient/client. To make confident estimates of the benefits of the new care regimen the nurse, along with health care colleagues and the patient/client themselves, needs to evaluate its effectiveness and efficacy.

The five key steps outlined above are not straightforward for clinical nurses. Some nurse graduates have been educated and supported in the research process by experienced researchers, either through undertaking a supervised research degree, or by membership of an experienced research team.

Most nurses have not had the opportunity to gain these experiences (Courtney, Rickard, Vickerstaff and Court, 2005, pp.6-10). For nurses steeped in the tradition and ethos of established expertise, the notion that set procedures may not be based on robust evidence, or that new knowledge may challenge established beliefs, may cause some discomfort. Furthermore, if busy nurses are required to make time to access the evidence base and update their knowledge and practice, there are human and financial resource implications. At a time of staff shortages and difficulties with staff recruitment and retention, meeting the government mandate regarding evidence-based practice can seem insurmountable. Under these circumstances, nurses need a range of support mechanisms to engage in evidence-based practice (Pearson and Craig, 2002, pp.10-12).

Resources available to review evidence-based practice

For nurses unfamiliar with standard research procedures, accessing reviews of the best available evidence for nursing practices can be most helpful. This is greatly facilitated by easy access to health care information through the internet. Electronic portals such as Google and databases such as MEDLINE have increased accessibility to a range of information for general inquiry, education, research and clinical practice. With the current emphasis on evidence-based practice and clinical governance, it has become mandatory for all health professionals to carry out electronic searches of what constitutes best practice. In many countries competencies for practice require that health staff is able to demonstrate evidence-based practice. Considerable infrastructure has been developed to support this aim including, for example, the National Institute for Clinical Excellence in the UK, the Agency for Health Care Research and Quality in the USA, and in Australia the National Institute for Clinical Studies (NICS) (NHS Executive 2001).

Clinical effectiveness literature can be obtained from a wide range of publications, databases and organisations. As already identified, the internet can provide access to a wide range of information sources, some of which has been critically evaluated. Journals can be located via the internet to obtain useful and up-to-date information on research evidence. The Journal of Evidence-Based Nursing is one such journal providing a range of peer-reviewed research articles aimed at keeping nurses abreast of important advances in nursing interventions and outcomes. The Open Nursing Journal is a freely-available, peer-reviewed journal which aims to provide the most complete and reliable source of information on current developments in nursing, and is indexed in PubMed Central, the PubMed Directory of Open Access H Journals, Open J-Gate and Journal/Seek. Digests such as Effective Health Care (website: www.york.ac.uk/in

st/crd/em.htm) provide short summaries of research evidence referenced to enable follow-ups of any areas of particular interest. Professional associations can also be important sources of grey literature and tend to specialise in evidence-based information.

These databases greatly increase the accessibility of evidence with which to inform quality nursing practice. However, when considering the evidence accessed it is important to evaluate the quality and applicability of this evidence to particular situations and for different health settings. Critical appraisal of the research conducted is needed to ensure the recommendations arising are based on sound evidence (Kitson, Rycroft-Malone, Harvey et al., 2008). While all studies ought to demonstrate rigour in study methodology and be based on the design most suitable in answering the study questions, there are differences in the review procedures for qualitative, quantitative and mixed methods studies. Having access to a range of methodological checklists can greatly assist the process of evaluating different types of studies. Electronic copies of these checklists can be found at www.salford.uk/hcprdu/assessment.htm.

Accessing expert reviews of evidence-based practice

These databases are an excellent resource for nurses, however, evaluating the quality of the sourced literature can be daunting. To do this, nurses need to acquire the skills for systematically appraising and employing research evidence for clinical decision-making. This requires training and/or the support of experienced researchers and since critical appraisal requires some skill a three-pronged process is suggested: assessment of the quality of a study, assessment of the applicability of a study and interpretation of the study results for the individual patient within a particular context (Newman and Roberts, 2002, pp.109-19). For example, to determine the best way to evaluate a nursing intervention aimed at reducing unmet-need behaviour in persons with dementia, the nurse would need to understand the relative benefits of conducting a randomised control trial compared with a case study design (Chenoweth, King, Jeon, Brodaty, Stein-Parbury, Haas and Luscombe, 2009). On the other hand, if nurses are interested to know whether the older person's self-reported feelings predict depression, they will need to recognise that a cross-sectional study design is a suitable approach. To assist nurses in this conceptually daunting process, nurses are advised to access evidence-based reviews of studies on a topic of interest, such as those reported by the Cochrane Collaboration. The quality of the evidence in these reviews has already been evaluated by expert reviewers, including, for example, the advantages of restraint-free care in dementia (Ibrahim, Koch, Holland and Howie, 2009, pp.129-126).

The major institutes for supporting evidence-based practice in Australia are the National Institute of Clinical Studies (NICS) and the Joanna Briggs Institute for Evidence-Based Nursing (JBI). The NICS aims to improve health care by reporting the best-available evidence to reduce the implementation of non-evidence-based practice, i.e. to reduce the evidence-practice gap (Silagy, 2001). The NICS works with health staff in a series of consultation rounds to identify gaps in practice that are considered to be widespread, clinically significant and needing urgent change. A nursing reference group was established in 2002 to include their voices in eviden-cepractice gaps in nursing. Major projects have focused on pressure ulcer management and pain management in cancer patients. The NICS pressure ulcer resource guide can be located at ww w.nicsl.com.au. The NICS' clinical priority areas use change methodology to facilitate changes in routine practice and to foster the training of clinical champions to enable necessary evidence-based practice.

The JBI was established in 1996, and conducts primary research, systematic literature reviews and meta-analyses of research evidence of nursing practice. The institute also utilises evidence through implementation projects and the Practical Application of Clinical Evidence System. Nurses will find this service invaluable when searching for fact sheets on evidence-based best-practice in a wide range of nursing interventions (see http://www.joannabrigg

s.edu.au/pubs/best_practice.php). The Joanna Briggs Collaboration is a coordinated effort by a group of self-governing collaborating centres coordinated through the leadership by JBI.

Another valuable resource for nurse managers is the Evidence Check Review conducted by the Sax Institute in partnership with NSW Health. This independent Australian not-for-profit organisation improves health and health services by enabling the use of research in policy-making. Comprehensive reviews comprise detailed syntheses of relevant research evidence relating to a defined research question. The Institute facilitates reviews of existing research and evidence tailored to the individual needs of the health agency (www.saxinstitute.org.au).

Nursing is at its best when practice embodies an awareness of the outcomes that are most important to the patient/client. Best-practice guidelines should strive to achieve this end by anticipating the range of clinical scenarios, outcomes of care and patient/client and family preferences (Osbourne and Webster, 2005, pp.185-9). Therefore, guidelines for nursing practice are developed with the aim of identifying the best way to serve patients/clients, with three key elements guiding their development: they must deal with defined clinical situations; best practice must be the ultimate aim; and rigorously applied proven methods must be employed in identifying quality care practices (Institute of Medicine Committee to Advise the Public Health Service on Practice

Guidelines, 1990). In Australia the National Health and Medical Research Council (NHMRC) (1999) has incorporated key qualities into nine guiding principles for effective guideline development. The nine principles are grouped under six requirements: validity and reproducibility; representativeness; flexibility and adaptability; cost-effectiveness; reliability; and applicability. The web source for these guideline principles is www.health.gov.au/nhmrc/publications/ophome.htm. Practice guidelines meeting these requirements can assist nurses in selecting those with a very high standard of evidence, reflecting the quintessential expression of the integrity of the profession.

Despite the usefulness of evidence-based guidelines for practice nurses, many nurses may not employ them to improve or guide care and thus provide the optimal conditions for care quality. A number of factors have been identified, including: the interest and willingness of nurses to implement these guidelines; the complexity of the guidelines and ease of implementation; the requirement to have specific resources for implementation; the health status of patients, especially those with complex needs and presence of co-morbidities; and insufficient organisational support (Francke, Smit, de Veer and Mistiaen, 2008). A recommendation from this research is that multiple approaches are needed to convince nurses that evidence-based clinical guidelines are important to improve the quality and consistency of nursing practice. These approaches might include educational interventions, audits and other actions for nursing improvement. A recommended strategy includes making available the evidence that supports the efficacy of employing particular clinical guidelines (Francke, Smit, de Veer and Mistiaen, 2008, pp.44-7).

A useful database of evidence-based patient/client outcomes signalling nursing practice success is the Nursing Outcomes Classification (NOC), developed as a comprehensive and standardised classification of patient/client outcomes that are responsive to nursing interventions (Moorhead, Johnson and Maas, 2004). Seven domains of outcome have been identified and classified into: functional health; physiological health; psychosocial health; health knowledge and behaviour; perceived health; family health; and community health. Core outcomes sensitive to nursing care include: ambulation; comfort; communication ability; health promoting behaviour; knowledge of disease process, self-care and health status, nutritional status, pain levels and disruptive effects; participation in health care decisions; and safety behaviour such as falls prevention, self-care and tissue integrity. Each of these topic areas offers important information to guide nursing care of the older person, since they are based on strong evidence of planned and positive patient/client outcomes (Moorhead, Johnson and Maas, 2004).

An extension of this classification system for evidence-based nursing care is the International Classification of Nursing Practice (INCP), which provides a system for classifying patient/client outcomes responsive to nursing intervention, as well as categorising these phenomena and nursing actions. The ICNP (2004) was developed to provide a common language for describing nursing practice in order to improve communication among nurses and with other health professionals. Nursing outcomes are referred to in this classification system as results in relation to nursing problems or diagnoses that are measured over time. Website: www.icn.ch/icnpupdate.htm#Intro.

Examples of evidence-based nursing in practicein aged care

There are many examples in the literature of nursing-sensitive health outcomes for older people and health systems. The following outlines a small number of nursing-led studies in the area of aged care that have resulted in improved patient/client and family carer outcomes, improved care practice and health systems and informed health and aged care policy.

Health promotion and self-care

A health outcome measure suitable for use with older people was developed by Resnick et al. (2001), based on the theory of self-efficacy for self-management (Bandura, 1995). The study focused on the influence of expectations about exercise and actual participation in exercise for community-dwelling older people. In this study community nurses employed self-efficacy theory to develop an instrument for measuring the older person's interest and engagement in health exercise programs and to test the outcomes. The result of this research was the development of the Outcome Expectation for Exercise (OEE) Scale for Use in Older Adults (Resnick et al., 2001). This tool is a valuable aid for nurses when measuring the older person's willingness and readiness to engage in exercise programs for health maintenance and when recovering from illness and disability (Chang, 2005, p.121).

Employing self-efficacy theory with 400 older people experiencing either heart failure, chronic respiratory disease, Parkinson's disease or long-term schizophrenia, Australian nurses Gallagher, Donoghue, Chenoweth and Stein-Parbury (2008) investigated the role of self-efficacy in self-care for these chronic illness groups. Since chronic diseases are common among older people and cannot be cured, they need to be managed well to achieve quality of life (McCormack, 2009, pp.30-33). Self-efficacy theory posits that optimal self-management requires the person with chronic illness to be knowledgeable about the condition and related treatment, able to participate in decision-making concerning health management and willing to perform health-related activities (Bandura, 1995). These activities include taking prescribed medicines correctly, monitoring signs and symptoms and taking action when symptoms worsen, as well as making and keeping medical/health appointments. Self-efficacy is the confidence that a person has in their capability to plan and carry out behaviours to manage the situation in the best possible way (Holman and Lorig, 1992). Gallager, Donoghue, Chenoweth and Stein-Parbury (2008) showed that self-efficacy had a positive influence on self-management for the four chronic illness groups. This is an important finding because self-efficacy may be one of the few factors predictive of self-management that is amenable to nursing influence through education, guidance and support.

Another area of nursing research that has led to improved understanding and health promotion for a vulnerable group is stress associated with the role of carer. An early study by Bowers (1987) investigated the impact of the role of carer with a view to identifying the purvey of all activities involved in caring for an older relative/friend, and also to identify aspects that were protective and non-protective of the carer's health and wellbeing. Bowers found that even when an older relative/friend is located to a residential care facility the carer continues to provide care while the sense of burden of care is not necessarily reduced. A new type of care emerges where the carer attempts to preserve the identity and individuality of their relative/friend. These concepts were tested with a large number of carers in Sweden (Eckwall, Swiberg and Hallberg, 2004) in which the researchers identified that carers engaged in a range of protective care activities to maintain reciprocity in the relationship between themselves and the person being cared for. These activities changed over time as the caring role became more demanding. This research has led to the development of an explanatory model of care-giving that more easily identifies potential areas of carer stress and satisfaction with this role, with hopes that it will provide timely education and support to prevent burnout by encouraging reciprocity and satisfaction (Nolan, Lundh, Grant et al., 2003).

Improved health outcomes

As the health clinicians most readily able to assess and meet the needs of older people in a range of health settings, nurses are in the best position to reduce iatrogenic illness occurring in this vulnerable group. Delirium, falls, pressure ulcers, dehydration, constipation and de-conditioning are largely preventable and amenable to skilled nursing care. Important research has been conducted by nurses aiming to prevent these avoidable health outcomes, for example, the work in delirium assessment and management by Inouye and colleagues (2005). In order to assist health staff differentiate confusion in delirium from other confused states and thus protect the older patient from serious ill-health and possible death, Inouye's team conducted a number of well-controlled research studies with older patients between 1990 and 2005. This body of research resulted in the development of a validated delirium measure, the Confusion Assessment Method (CAM) (Inouye, Leo-Summers, Zhang et al., 2005), which provides nurses and other health staff with a standardised way to accurately detect delirium in a range of settings. Employing this tool, a group of Australian nurse researchers facilitated a redesign of nursing care practice (Day, Higgins and Koch, 2009). The study showed an improvement in delirium assessment for older hospital patients, prevention of delirium for a large number of patients and implementation of more effective delirium and management strategies. These positive outcomes were sustained at a 12 month follow-up.

A study conducted in acute care settings by Parker, Fadayevantan and Lee (2006) revealed that the implementation of evidence-based practice can help avoid some serious outcomes for older patients, such as functional impairment, cognitive decline and altered physiology, which may render patients vulnerable to multiple problems, like pressure ulcers. Another serious outcome for older patients that is amenable to improved nursing practice is an adverse drug event. In a US-based study of 15,000 older patients in 2000, 64% of patients over 65 years of age experienced a preventable drug event (Thomas and Brennan, 2000). Similar findings have occurred in Australian research, revealing that prevention of negative drugrelated effects, such as falls, can occur by implementing skilled nursing care. This can be achieved by following best-practice guidelines, including conducting comprehensive sensory, cognitive and health assessment, falls-risk assessment, vigilant patient monitoring, patient and staff education and paying attention to the physical and psychosocial needs of older patients (Dempey, 2004).

Aiming to improve outcomes for aged care residents with dementia through a nursing care intervention, Chenoweth, King, Jeon, Brodaty, Stein-Parbury, Haas and Luscombe (1999) conducted a cluster-randomised controlled trial of Person-Centred Care (PCC) and Dementia Care Mapping (DCM) and compared it with usual nursing care practices (UC). Fifteen care sites were randomly allocated to PCC, DCM and UC and a wide range of outcomes were measured, including resident wellbeing, quality of life, behaviours associated with dementia, restraint use, accidents, injuries and hospitalisation related to resident behaviour and nursing practice quality. The results of this trial concluded that both PCC and DCM significantly reduced agitation-related behaviour such as pacing, perseveration and calling out (vocalisation), and changed eating and sleep patterns, when compared with UC. Wellbeing improved and falls were reduced for residents in the DCM homes. PCC was the most cost-effective nursing approach for this client group. These results confirm conclusions drawn in previous PCC and DCM research (for example, Brooker 2005; Fossey, Ballard and Juszczak, 2006) and support results of a comprehensive review of non-pharmacological interventions for the management of dementia-related behaviour (Cohen-Mansfield, Libin and Marx, 2007). These positive findings justify the superior benefits of individually tailored nursing management approaches for persons with dementia, compared with drug treatment and standard distraction techniques.

In the older hospital patient population, malnutrition and dehydration are common occurrences. Duncan et al. (2006) found that maintaining good hydration and nutrition can be achieved through understanding the limitations of the older person during a hospital admission and responding to these limitations through supplemental feeding, assisting them with meals and fluids and ensuring staff are allocated protected time in which to assist the person maintain hydration and nutrition. Nurses can have a profound positive influence on the outcomes for older people in all health settings, but it is the acute care setting where this is most obvious. A good example is in the older person's preparation for safe hospital discharge, which should commence as soon as the patient's immediate treatment has commenced (Hickman, Phillip Newton and Halcombe, 2007). Comprehensive and regular assessment of the older person's functional, sensory and cognitive status are essential requirements to prevent iatrogenic illness and an unnecessarily lengthy hospital stay, both of which influence the older person's discharge readiness and destination (Care of Older Australian Working Group, (COOAWG) 2004). The argument for implementing evidence-based nursing care is strongly supported by these research findings.

A nursing-led study conducted with 98 nurse managers from 42 Japanese hospitals clearly revealed a direct relationship between nursing hours, restraint use and pressure ulcer development in older patients with dementia (Ibe, Ishizaki, Oku, Ota, Takabatake, Iseda, Ishikawa and Ueda, 2008). The study was stimulated by a growing concern about the critical shortage of Registered Nurses in Japan, the increasing numbers of older people being hospitalised for medical and social reasons and the growing incidence of poor patient outcomes. The total number of pressure ulcers occurring in the 87 care units over a three month period was 440, indicating a high rate of incidence for this population group. Increased use of physical restraint occurred for patients needing greater assistance with activities of daily living. The incidence of physical restraint use and pressure ulcers increased with decreases in numbers of Registered Nurses. These findings align with the perceptions of a large number of Australian Registered Nurses (Duffield et al., 2008) that a reduction in Registered Nurse hours reduces care quality and patient outcomes.

Retaining skilled nurses in aged care

Reduced numbers of Registered Nurses are widespread throughout the Australian health and aged care sectors. A systematic literature review conducted by Chenoweth, Jeon, Merlyn and Brodaty (2009) scanned 226 international research papers on nurse recruitment and retention. One hundred and five papers relevant to recruitment and retention strategies for dementia and aged care nursing were selected for closer examination. Of these, 25 papers were rated at level 2++ to 3, according to the guidelines of the National Institute for Health and Clinical Excellence (NICE, 2006). These 25 critically reviewed papers revealed that combined, rather than single, factors are more effective in nurse recruitment and retention. The research literature makes clear that dementia and aged care nursing demand a great deal of investment in the nurse's emotional wellbeing and building up of their professional role. Consequently, these nurses say they need to be supported and nurtured, professionally and personally, in order to consider entering and remaining in the specialty. As well, a career choice in the specialty is only attractive and successful when that commitment is adequately rewarded in a range of ways. Poor remuneration for work that requires quite high levels of skill and commitment, particularly parity with other sectors, was a common theme of dissatisfaction for aged and dementia care nurses. However, these nurses value the intrinsic rewards of nursing work and assert that their concern lies more with the way lower pay diminishes their status and professional respect. Family-friendly policy rated highly in nurses' decisions to remain employed, particularly in a sector dominated by women, with flexibility in schedules and a healthy work-life balance considered essential. Specialised training, particularly for skills of leadership and teamwork, along with adequate staffing levels to redress the sector's ubiquitous overload and unpaid overtime, are the next most important factors and necessary conditions for job satisfaction and retention (Chenoweth, Jeon, Merlyn and Brodaty, 2009). The findings of this evidence-based literature review signal that job 'embeddedness' is central to retaining nursing staff, evidenced by a culture of openness and respect that facilitates communication and in turn encourages a flatter hierarchy among staff who have a higher level of discretion in their practice and greater work-life balance. These factors lead to more satisfaction and effective commitment, both necessary components for implementing quality nursing care. The evidence elicited in this review provides health service providers and managers with some clear directions for improving aged care nurse retention.

Service quality

The Aged Care Structural Reform Package of 1997 has profoundly influenced policy within the Australian aged care sector, most notably ageing-in-place, a new aged care resident classification instrument and service standard. To investigate whether these structural characteristics directly influenced service quality and resident outcomes, Richardson and Bartlett (2009) employed Donabedian's (1980) model for exploring the determinants of quality service. All residential aged care services in Queensland, Australia, provided facility accreditation outcome reports for analysis in a time series design over six years. Trends in high and low care facilities, standards of compliance and changing care categories for residents were analysed to explore changes over time. The findings indicated that ageing-in-place facilities provided progressively more care for more dependent residents and had the highest compliance ratings on all accreditation standards. These outcomes reveal that ageing-in-place facilities were successful in building capacity to provide care for more dependent residents. There are important national policy implications arising from this research, notably staffing ratios and skill-mix requirements, standards of care quality and infrastructure requirements to assist aged care facilities to transition to ageing-in-place homes.

Measuring the quality of care services is still in its infancy, given the complex structures, processes and outcomes that comprise health service reviews (Donabedian, 1988). In Australia many government-sanctioned bodies have attempted to improve care services through accreditation processes, for example the Australian Residential Aged Care Services Accreditation Agency. A few Australian nurse researchers have been working on developing instruments to assess quality of care within the residential aged care sector (e.g. Burke, Chenoweth and Stein-Parbury, 2009). The Clinical Care Indicators' measure (Courtney et al., 2007) provides a step forward for the residential aged care sector. The tool has been developed through an iterative research process, tested in Australian residential aged care homes, and is currently being benchmarked to allow for wider use in health care settings. This and other quality measures being developed and tested by nurse-led teams will ultimately elevate nursing practice standards in health and aged care.

Conclusion

The overwhelming case for employing evidence-based nursing practice is that it leads to positive outcomes for patients/clients and families, but also can improve care standards and health systems' standards and inform health policy. While it is unrealistic that the majority of nurses will engage in research to achieve these ends, they should integrate research evidence and professional experience to guide their practice. The difficulty for nurses, as discussed earlier in this chapter, is their unfamiliarity with interpreting and applying research evidence in practice. Accessing evidence-based guidelines for practice will greatly assist them; however, they still need help with implementing best-practice and evaluating the effects. An innovative model called TEAM (Translating Evidence into Aged Care Methods) has been developed by a team of Australian nurse researchers and clinicians to assist nurses to better understand how to engage in evidence-based nursing (Winbolt, Nay and Featherstonhough, 2009, pp.447-9).

TEAM is founded on the philosophy of the link between leadership and learning, and employs a multidisciplinary team approach to implement best-practice guidelines through change principles of action research and grounded theory data sampling and analysis. The approach is familiar to nurses who have undertaken efforts towards continuous quality improvement; however, the action methodology employed serves as an educative and empowering process. This innovative process has the potential to overcome some of the barriers that inhibit implementation of evidence-based nursing, notably through the professional collaboration encouraged in seeking better health and health care practices.

Chapter 7

Person-centred care in aged care

Catherine Brown, RN, PGrad. Dip. Psych. Of Old Age, MN (Aged Care)
Project Officer, Psychogeriatric Service, Department of Health and Families, NT Government;
previously Senior Manager, Benevolent Society, Sydney, NSW

Objectives:

This chapter will enable the reader to:

1) Demonstrate an understanding of the concept of personcentred care;
2) Explain the relationship between codes of professional conduct and codes of ethics and personhood;
3) Describe and discuss the psychosocial impact of illness on an older person living alone in the community;
4) Demonstrate the ability to identify the principles that underpin clinical and moral decision-making; and
5) Formulate a care plan for an older person admitted to an orthopaedic or rehabilitation ward with

a fractured neck of femur using a person centred approach.

Introduction

Person-centred care is based on a social paradigm encompassing the notion that nurses should focus on the strengths of the older person and the uniqueness of the individual, especially those with cognitive impairment, thus maintaining their identities while simultaneously providing them with a sense of dignity and self-esteem. Concepts of person-centred relationships in education and counselling and between community members were developed by Rogers in the late 20th Century (Rogers, 2008). Kitwood (1997) initiated much discussion on the person-centred care approach in dementia care by defining personhood and relating it to positive person work and decreasing the influence of malignant social psychology (Kitwood, 1997; DeBellis, Bradley, Wotherspoon, Walter, Guein, Cecchin and Peterson, 2009). His focus was to promote relationships between the person with dementia, or any vulnerable person, and their carer, upholding respect and trust and avoiding negative overtures which may intimidate, stigmatise, disempower and infantilise people. Table 3 indicates the connection between personhood and person-centred care and highlights the significance of mutual respect within relationships and within a social context (McCormack, 2004).

Table 3. Person-centred care and personhood

Concepts of person-centred care	Link with Kitwood's definition of personhood
Being in relation with other people	People exist in relationships
Being in social world	People are social beings
Being in place	People have a context through which their personhood is articulated
Being with self	Being recognised, respected and trusted as a person impacts on a person's sense of self

Core elements of person-centred care

It is difficult to isolate a definition for both person-centred care and personhood. Much of the literature calls person-centred care an 'approach' rather than a model, thus allowing authors to suggest various components of such an approach and its key features that may be included in a discussion on the subject (e.g. providing social and sensory stimulation and working with people's beliefs and values). Key words used to describe person-centred care consistently include holistic, whole person, advocacy, empowerment, relationships, trust and respect. It is therefore the basis of what we do and how we do it that helps to provide an outcome of care that does not leave a person feeling devalued, humiliated and worthless.

The German philosopher Kant in 1784 described personhood as the foundation on which ethical principles are built (Thompson, Melia, and Boyd, 2000; Kitwood, 1997; McCormack, 2003). He postulated that all individuals have the right to be respected and that the key to respecting others lies at the acceptance of a person's autonomy. Nurses in Australia and New Zealand are bound by professional codes of conduct developed by the Australian Nursing and Midwifery Council (ANMC, 2008) and the Nursing Council of New Zealand (NCNZ, 2008). Additionally, the International Council of Nurses (ICN, 2006) *Code of Ethics for Nurses* identifies core ethical principles which guide nurses' practice and decision-making. In the preamble, the ICN code states that 'inherent in nursing is respect for human rights, including cultural rights, the right to life and choice, to dignity and to be treated with respect'(p1). The ANMC developed the *Code of Ethics for Nurses in Australia (ANMC, 2008)* which relates to the ICN position statements and, along with national competency standards, provides the framework for professional practice for nurses in Australia.

These codes all refer to professional practices that embrace a culture of respect for the person in their care, nurturing dignity, values, beliefs and ethnicity, in addition to supporting and promoting patients' physical and emotional wellbeing. Thompson, Melia and Boyd (2000) describe the leap forward nursing has achieved in developing ethical frameworks that underpin the very nature of care delivery, nursing management and the broad structure on which the profession is built. They detail economic, demographic and social changes that have necessitated debate within the nursing profession to ensure that nurses are supported in clinical and moral judgements related to patient-centred care.

Person-centred care and older adults

Older people are a vulnerable group in society. The ANMC Conduct Statement 8 describes the centrality of trusting relationships in nursing care and acknowledges the power differential between the nurse and the people in their care, in whichever health setting nurses practice. Many old people have undergone multiple losses, whether physical, emotional or cognitive, and as such are at risk of losing their self-identity and the ability and confidence to make their own health care decisions (Allan and Killick, 2008). This is more evident in the person experiencing a dementing illness but may also be seen in frail and isolated elderly and in older adults generally.

Commonly, throughout the nurses' codes, the themes of respect and patients' rights are emphasised. Key principles of personcentred care include acknowledging and respecting the uniqueness of the individual. This encompasses their social, psychological and physiological differences, and by upholding positive interactions and core practices of nurturing and advocacy, these fundamental rights will be acknowledged. Additionally, underlying principles in the New Zealand Ministry of Health

Guidelines and Strategies (New Zealand Ministry of Health, 2004; 2002b) also dictate these core philosophies with a strong emphasis on restorative care and the empowerment of the older person to make well informed decisions.

The Best Practice Guidelines Project, Toronto, 'Shaping the Future of Nursing' (Registered Nurses Association of Toronto, 2002), defines person- or client-centred care as *'an approach in which clients are viewed as whole persons; it is not merely about delivering services where the client is located. Client centre care involves advocacy, empowerment, and respecting the client's autonomy, voice, self-determination, and participation in decision-making'.* The key focus of the guideline is the promotion of independence and maximisation of health outcomes through empowerment and a psycho-social approach to care practices. This model is promoted through e-learning packages supported by the Registered Nurses Association, Toronto.

If nurses undertook to wholly embrace the professional codes of ethics and professional behaviour, contemporary health care practice that currently detracts from a patient's personhood could be transformed to adopt practices that support a person's rights, values, beliefs and abilities to make informed decisions that promote wellness. Furthermore, the concept of person-centred care should be moved beyond the focus of the delivery of best practice dementia care to accommodate all older people in our care.

Relationships

A person-centred care approach usually requires support from family members and others who have significant relationships with older adults. This is particularly crucial in the acute care setting where older people present in a frail state and often with complex disease states (Nolan, 2006; Kilshaw, 2009).

Kitwood's work emphasised the importance of people (e.g. the nurse and person with dementia) making a mutual connection (or 'connectivity') with each other (e.g. through body language, empathy etc.) in order to support the person with dementia in their ability to have some level of communication with others. Moreover, the key to preserving a person's 'self ' lies in information sharing by the older person and mutual respect between them and care workers for each person's traditions and values. Current evidence demonstrates the need for a comprehensive and informative assessment and history from an older person presenting to hospital in order to improve discharge planning and reduce the risk of re-admission or deleterious health events while an in-patient (Nolan, 2006; Kilshaw, 2009; Lim, Cong, Caplan and Gray, 2009).

Furthermore, recent research (McCormack, 2003; McCormack and McCance, 2006) suggests that older people's expectations of health care institutions include being treated as individuals, that nurses would act as advocates and that relationships with health professionals would be underpinned by trust and a sharing of knowledge.

Enhanced communication and relationship building skills are key factors in a person-centred care model (Allan and Killick, 2008; Grosch, Medvene and Woolcott, 2008). The social world of the older person may be heavily dependent on relationships and may be influenced by historical issues (e.g. untimely death of a young family member, financial hardship, environmental adversities or perhaps misfortunes related to past life decisions), and the nurse must demonstrate resourcefulness in determining the dimensions of relationships that may affect a patient's wellbeing. Additionally, illness often creates an imbalance or a change in a relationship and the nurse must be alert to these dynamics to ensure that information (e.g. taking a nursing history) is comprehensive and non-judgemental and is not likely to result in poor decisions or lead to ageist interpretations.

In order to enhance health care outcomes for the older person an environment of shared communication should be initiated from the commencement of caregiving. The older person may have specific impairments that will inhibit clear communication, but may also be experiencing acute anxiety or be preoccupied with their current environment, which will impact on their ability to think clearly and participate fully in the initial assessment (McCormack, 2003; Thompson,

Girling, Green and Wai, 2008; Moehead, Barraclough and Alvai, 2008). This might occur, for instance, when a client is interviewed by a community care case manager, on entry to a residential care facility, or on presentation to a hospital department. The nurse, therefore, must ensure that sufficient time is allocated to the initial assessment. Early intervention that includes comprehensive history taking, an understanding of cultural beliefs and practices and an assessment and understanding of physical and cognitive limitations will assist in building a relationship based on reciprocity and trust. Additionally, this will improve the capacity to provide appropriate care in an appropriate environment. It is good practice to seek validation of information given by the older person by discussing results of assessments (for instance, with the client or the person responsible) prior to developing their care plan and ensuring that mutually acceptable interpretations and health goals have been identified.

Studies conducted in aged care facilities have shown that successful person-centred care has been embraced by administrators and care workers who have a focus on developing good relationships with their residents and families. They commonly acknowledge residents' preferences and value input from all their consumers including residents, family members, guardians, visitors, contractors and visiting health professionals, as well as all employees (Fisher and Wallhagen, 2008; Walent and Kayser-Jones, 2008). Alternatively, paucity of appropriate resources including specialist aged care clinical nurse consultants, poor knowledge of ageing and aged care and lack of empathy for the older person have been shown to contribute to adverse outcomes for older people in hospital.

Advocacy in the acute care setting for older adults

The nurse as advocate puts forward an argument or statement on someone else's behalf, representing their client and pursuing the interests or rights of that person. In an acute care ward this may, for example, be the nurse who contacts the community care program to ensure services are booked for commencement post-discharge. Acting on the patient's behalf, the nurse advocates, on behalf of the patient, for an extension of the inpatient stay, reducing the risk of an untoward health event occurring in the gap period post-discharge and prior to community service follow-up provision. Communication pathways between ward staff and discharge planners, along with collaborative multidisciplinary teamwork, will ensure that the focus of the health outcome is on the individual, not on the event (Lim, Cong, Caplan, and Gray, 2009).

Another example may be where the timing of a physiotherapy program conflicts with the administration of analgesia. Evidence-based practice in pain management indicates that an older person's ability to cope with an exercise session is enhanced by timely administration of analgesia. Ensuring the older person understands the importance of this approach and communicating to allied health staff is a preferred outcome instead of dismissing the exercise session due to complaints of pain and discomfort.

More broadly, however, and in the framework of a personcentred approach in an acute care setting, the nurse is confronted by situations requiring advocacy and related decision-making on a daily basis. The professional codes of conduct uphold the right of patients to advocacy and the expectation of nurses to be responsible and to 'promote and protect the interests of people receiving treatment and care' (Conduct Statement 4, ANMC, 2008). As previously discussed, care decisions are based on multiple sources including accurate history taking, comprehensive assessments, evidence-based practice and, importantly, client preferences. An important role nurses must incorporate into their practice is assisting older people and their families to understand the evidence and the risks and consequences related to clinical intervention and client decisions (McCormack and McCance, 2006; Ibrahim, Koch, Holland and Howie, 2009; Conn, Burks, Rantz and Knusen, 2002).

Case study #1

Mrs Cumming is a 79 year old woman and has been transferred to the medical ward following 20 hours in the Emergency Department. She has a diagnosis of pneumonia and swollen (L) knee following a fall at home. She has no support person with her at the time of transfer. Her treatment orders include intravenous antibiotics, p.r.n. analgesia and physiotherapy for her chest and knee. Mrs Cumming is quiet, has not received any analgesia and has been incontinent. Consider factors that may impede Mrs Cumming's recovery. What assessments would you consider are needed to be undertaken to assist her recovery? At what stage would you discuss discharge planning and what considerations should be taken into account?

Assessment and care planning and person-centred care

In examining the forces that impact on nurses' ability to deliver person-centred care in any health care setting, the literature (Nolan, 2006; Ibrahim et al., 2009; Conn et al., 2002) indicates the following barriers:

- Inconsistent staffing
- Organisational policies and practices
- Physical environment
- Lack of knowledge
- Lack of communication
- Ageist attitudes of staff

Recent discussions to promote person-centred care in the acute setting highlight the significance of good working relationships within an organisation, in particular those workplaces where innovative practice and decision-making are encouraged (McCormack, 2003; Fleming and Kayser-Jones, 2008). Increased education relevant to respectful communication with the elderly by all hospital staff, increased awareness of the impact of the hospital environment on an older person and an understanding of the benefits of detailed assessments and history taking will in time provide a shift away from ageist attitudes. Considering the complex factors influencing illness in the older person, it is important to undertake detailed assessments to complete the most accurate picture of what the older person is experiencing, and to identify iatrogenic risk factors. Additionally, environmental audits of acute care wards and aged care facilities should be designed to identify stimuli that have negative impacts on older people, such as poor signage that reduces their independence and increases their confusion, or unsuitable low chairs or lounges that restrict their ability to transfer independently and safely.

Table 4. Acute care barriers to recovery

Negative contributing factors to recovery	Considerations
Pain	Assessments using validated tools (e.g. Abbey Pain Scale, PAIN Aid (for cognitively impaired)) Is sleep disturbed? Are mobility aids adequate?

Negative contributing factors to recovery	Considerations
Poor nutrition	Is seating/positional placement in bed enabling the patient? Consider impeding equipment (e.g. IV fluids) Can they open packaging? Or feed themselves?
Sensory impairment	Assess abilities, Are sensory aids with patient?
Environment	Are bed rails impeding access to a toilet? Is the noise level of the ward causing distress?

Comprehensive interdisciplinary assessments are encouraged to ensure accurate diagnosis, realistic interventions that include physical and psychosocial factors and optimal outcomes. Current hospital health outcome reports highlight the numbers of older people in hospital beds with length of stays exceeding 30 days (Australian Institute of Health and Welfare, 2006). The complexity of the bio-psychological care model needed to attain positive health outcomes for older people is often overlooked. Even if it is considered, the model is often discarded due to lack of suitably trained staff to undertake thorough assessments, poor geriatric knowledge and short-term priorities as opposed to long-term goals (e.g. increasing bed turnover statistics without considering re-admission rate, reduced health care expenditure (Lim et al., 2009; Moehead et al., 2008)).

The advantage of the interdisciplinary approach to assessment and management is regulated team discussions within a case management model that enhances communication between the client and the various medical and allied health staff and reduces the impact of exhaustive consultations between individual team members and the older patient (Thompson et al., 2008; Davis, Dorevitch and Garratt, 2009). Furthermore, the code of professional conduct (ANMC Conduct statement 7) emphasises the expectation that 'nurses support the health, wellbeing and informed decision-making of people requiring or receiving care'. Additionally, this statement enforces the responsibility of the nurse to act as an advocate to ensure their client has adequate representation if deemed necessary (Lim et al., 2009).

Care planning requires input from all members of the team as well as the patient and their significant others. Early intervention and pro-active discharge planning, along with consistent care support, will minimise obstacles that delay recovery (Lim et al., 2009). The following considerations will improve effective discharge planning from acute care:

- Identification at admission of psychosocial problems
- Working with patients' preferences
- Consultation with family members or significant others
- Assessment of current living conditions
- Assessment of risk of abuse
- Assessment of level of mobility
- Identification of community support (GP, pharmacist, community care provider) required

- Identification of personal care needs
- Identification of environmental aids
- Medication management and review
- Identification of nutrition needs
- Ability to manage finances
- Sensory impairment
- Assessment of risk of falls
- Working with existing social supports to reduce the risk of isolation

Person-centred care in residential care settings

Studies reviewing attitudes of care workers in aged care facilities confirm that an overall culture of person-centred care exists where staffing is consistent and resident advocacy programs are promoted (Fisher and Wallhagen, 2008; Walent and Kayser-Jones, 2008). An advocacy program may involve a system of allocation of residents to staff members who in turn become a spokesperson for that resident if and when needed. The staff member may then take steps to ensure that their residents' views are made known, for example, to the menu committee, or that they have the appropriate mobility aid or have access to a volunteer program for spiritual support (i.e., to take the older adult to church). They may also be allocated as the initial key contact for the family member when items of clothing need replacing or birthday gifts are being considered.

Additionally, analysis of the utilisation of the model of transactional leadership, where directors of nursing use consumer engagement (for example, with residents and their families) and staff mentoring programs, has shown that autonomy of the older person is more likely to be reinforced (Fleming and Kayser-Jones, 2008). Residential care settings where rosters are flexible to enable staffing movements to reflect current resident mix, and where the environment is able to be altered to suit the individual needs of residents, support a framework of person-centred care. Lounge chair settings that can be grouped to provide privacy or alternatively to enhance conversation create a homelike atmosphere that enhances dignity and promotes social interaction. Residents' bedrooms should reflect the personality and interests of the resident rather than resembling a modern hotel room. Environmental designs such as these also empower care staff to feel comfortable in using therapies and activities such as reminiscence or aromatherapy, where the focus of the home is a social approach rather than a medical model of care.

Conclusion

Current evaluations of models of service in the acute care sector have resulted in an increase in specialist geriatric services to enable early screening and improved case management along the care continuum. Models include an aged care triage nurse in accident and emergency departments, hospital and community clinical nurse consultants and nurse practitioners and specialist aged care wards (Thompson et al., 2008; Davis et al., 2009; Kilshaw, 2009; Moehead et al., 2008). These measures, which provide a foundation for good person-centred care, have been shown to reduce hospital stays, decrease the risk of re-admission and increase the likelihood that the older person will remain at home. For these reasons alone, Kitwood's creed of 'positive personhood', where the core values are to guard against clients being 'misunderstood, discounted, undermined, undervalued or disregarded', is inextricably reflected in the nurses' codes of ethics and professional conduct.

Reflective questions

1) Identify and reflect on a situation where a health outcome for an older person could have been improved by a person centred approach?
2) What do you understand by the term 'autonomy' as it relates to nursing an older person?
3) What is the difference between 'treatment', 'control' and 'care' as they relate to nursing practice?
4) Describe an area of conflict that occurred where an organisational policy impacted on an older person's choice.
5) Identify the Code of Ethics and Guide for Ethical Conduct for Residential Aged Care and the Charter of Residents Rights and consider the barriers to developing a personcentred framework while working within these guidelines.

6) How aged friendly are the hospital wards in which you have undertaken your clinical placement or in which you are currently working?

Useful resources

www.RNAO.org/bestpractices
http://dementia.uow.edu.au.understandingdementiacare
http://epubs.scu.edu.au/hahs-pubs/21

Chapter 8

Common health problems of old age

Sharon Wall, RN, RGeriN, DNE, BaHlth Sc., MPH
Director, Ageing and Caring P/L

Objectives

This chapter will enable the reader to:

1) Identify the ways in which disease and illness presents in older people;
2) Evaluate the wide ranging impact of illness on older people;
3) Value the importance of assessment in caring for older people with health issues;
4) Recognise the significance of multiple pathology and iatrogenesis for older clients; and
5) Describe the specific impact and management of the following for older person:
    a) Hypothermia and Hyperthermia
    b) Falls
    c) Osteoporosis, Arthritis, Osteoarthritis and Rheumatoid Arthritis
    d) Continence/Incontinence
    e) Diabetes

f) Cardiovascular disease/Coronary Heart Disease
g) Stroke
h) Visual Defects
i) Hearing loss
j) Common Cancers

Introduction

As people age, the incidence of some illnesses and diseases increases exponentially. That being so, it is important to continue to challenge the wide misconception that ageing is synonymous with illness and decline. This is often a situation self-perpetuated by older people who may also see ageing as illness and may not seek nor receive treatments and advice they deserve.

The awareness and understanding of some of the more common health conditions that may be a challenge in old age should ensure that preventative measures can be undertaken (more in keeping with a primary health model of care) as well as prompt and responsive treatments, if required.

It is important to frame the discussion of common illnesses in old age within a framework of health promotion and prevention. After all, the key to longevity is the absence of disease and the prevention of ill health.

Apart from illnesses and disease processes which have a specific significance to ageing, there are also underlying conditions and situations which are unique to the ageing process that may influence or further compound illness presentation and subsequent outcomes.

As we know the Australian and New Zealand populations are ageing rapidly. A consequence of this phenomenon is that older adults use more health care resources and experience conditions that often require more intensive and invasive treatment.

The presentation of illnesses and health problems in older people often has some unique qualities which differentiate it from presentation in a younger cohort.

Older people, particularly those requiring hospitalisation, are seldom hospitalised with one illness but often have a number of interacting signs and symptoms or multiple presentations which may complicate the assessment and diagnostic process.

Multiple pathology refers to the existence of more than one significant clinical problem. This often makes diagnosis more complex and has a cumulative impact more profound than the individual problems in isolation. An awareness of the impact of multiple pathology on older people is vital when undertaking assessment and diagnosis (Milton, James C.et al., p.606).

Iatrogenesis also contributes significantly to illness in older people. Research indicates that 36-58% of older adults suffer iatrogenic illness during hospitalisation.*

[* http://www.dhmc.org/dhmc-internet-upload/file_collection/Iatrogenesis.]

The word 'iatrogenic' comes from the Greek words 'iatros' meaning 'the healer or physician' and 'gennan' meaning 'as a product of ' or due to the doctor (Webster, 2008). Iatrogenesis refers to any unintended and untoward consequence of well-intended health care interventions. Cascade iatrogenesis is a series of adverse events triggered by initial medical or nursing interventions which initiate a cascade of decline. Iatrogenesis occurs most frequently among the oldest, most functionally impaired patients and those with a higher severity of illness upon admission. According to Francis (2009) older adults suffer more diagnostic complications, medication reactions, therapeutic mishaps and falls than younger patients.

Risk factors for iatrogenesis in older clients include aged-related changes, co-morbidity (multiple pathology) and atypical presentation of disease and illness. The reserves of elderly people are less than those of younger people, so the impact of iatrogenic injury is often greater (Iatrogenic Injury in Australia, 2001).

Health systems are often embedded in ageist beliefs and health care approaches often limit the true potential and capacity of older people. Hopefully, as models of care continue to change to reflect contemporary thinking regarding education and training, increased evidence-based practice and recognition of responsibilities of all health professionals and increased consumerism by older people themselves, these problems will become less evident.

Additionally, the increased interest in ageing that is apparent through various global longitudinal studies of ageing (see the Australian Longitudinal Study of Ageing*) will not only increase the understanding of common health problems affecting older people but will also influence the quality and consistency of care provided.

[* http://flinders.edu.au/socsci/fcas/alsa/alsa_home.cfm]

Common health problems of ageing

Identifying what is considered to be 'common' in terms of health care issues to do with ageing is complex as it may be influenced by a number of variables, including gender, ethnicity and socioeconomic status.

Historically, Aboriginal and Torres Strait Islanders have poorer health status and lower life expectancy in contrast to the general population. This has resulted in lower numbers of the population living beyond 65 years. For health planning purposes, Aboriginal and Torres Strait Islander people aged 50 years and older are included in the older population category, but this continues to be an issue of policy debate (Cotter et al., p.87).

The markedly lower health status of Indigenous Australians is deeply rooted in their substantial and pervasive social inequality. This social inequality is characterised by poverty and powerlessness, reflected across the age continuum in measures of education, employment, income and housing, and is a significant contributor to mental health and general health issues across the ageing spectrum (Broe, 2009).

Vast health inequalities persist across a number of ethnic groups, as is clear from differences in life expectancy at birth. For example, while Japan has the highest life expectancy in the world at 82.2 years, in several countries in Africa the figure is as much as 40 years lower. Within countries, health inequalities also have an impact on life expectancy. For example, in the USA higher socioeconomic groups can expect to live up to 20 years longer than those from lower socioeconomic groups (WHO, 2008).

As further evidence of the need to cater for non-English speaking Australians, the Australian Institute of Health and Welfare bulletin (AIHW, October, 2003), titled, 'A Picture of Diabetes in Overseas-born Australians', reports that proportionally more overseas-born people, (35%) report having diabetes. Among the groups with the highest prevalence of diabetes are Asian-born people. Those born in the Middle East also report a high prevalence of diabetes.

Some diseases of ageing are specifically related to gender, as would be obvious in the presentations of both prostate and breast cancer, both of which are further expanded upon within this chapter.

This chapter also identifies some of the more common health or health-related problems associated with ageing, particularly those that uniquely impact on older people. It is by no means an exhaustive presentation but aims to assist the practitioner with introductory information while motivating the reader to examine these issues further.

Thermoregulation syndromes – Hypothermia

Disease and illness presentations may be compounded by difficulties in thermoregulation in older people. The ageing process impacts on the body's ability to adapt to the cold temperatures. With ageing, the body becomes less efficient at shivering or at diverting blood away from the surface of the body. Additionally, there is generally less subcutaneous fat so there is less insulation to prevent heat loss (Merck Manual, 2004).

Initial symptoms of hypothermia develop slowly and the older adult may report feeling cold and more than likely will begin to shiver. However, by the time body temperature has fallen further (often with this initial sign missed) other signs and symptoms may develop including slowness of movement and slowness of speech.

When the body temperature is low, messages travel more slowly through the brain and the rest of the nervous system. Abnormal heart rhythms (arrhythmias) may occur. The heart also slows down and blood pressure falls. The kidneys make less urine and digestion slows because muscles in the digestive tract contract less. If body temperature falls below about

30°C, organs are likely to stop working altogether and death is likely. A diagnosis of hypothermia is made on the basis of a body temperature below 35°C, which is confirmed by the use of a special hypothermia thermometer (Redfern and Ross, 2006).

Treatment

Hypothermia is a medical emergency in older people. Recovery is subsequently dependent upon how long the person has been cold, how low the body temperature has fallen and the person's general health before hypothermia developed.

The first goal when hypothermia is suspected or diagnosed is to keep the person warm and dry so that body temperature does not fall further. The person is also kept immobile, because exertion may pump very cold blood from the extremities back to the heart and lead to further complications. Emergency treatment focuses on warming the person slowly but any additional problems such as cardiac arrhythmias will need to be simultaneously addressed (O'Neill, 2002).

Hyperthermia

Hyperthermia occurs when the core body temperature rises above 40°C. Older people are at risk because of their difficulty in thermoregulation, a consequence of ageing. The older person with hyperthermia will appear flushed and sweaty and will have skin which is hot to the touch. They will often complain of nausea and headache and appear listless. They may have increased respirations and be tachycardic, and will generally have a history of being exposed in some way to the sun for a prolonged time, or to some other type of heat source (Merck Manual, 2004).

Treatment

Treatment includes slowly decreasing the older adult's body temperature by providing cool fluids, removing restrictive clothing and tepid sponging if required. The nurse should continue to monitor outputs and temperature closely (Redfern and Ross, 2006).

Falls

There is an increased risk of falling with increasing age and research indicates that older people who have suffered a fall are at increased risk of falling again (Lord, et al., 2001). There is a high incidence of falls in residential aged care facilities (Lord, et al., 2001). Falls may result in injury which range from scratches and bruises to fractures and extreme events including major lacerations and cerebral events requiring hospitalisation. In Australia, an estimated one in three older persons living at home experience a fall annually (Older Australian at a Glance, 2007).

The following information from Hospitalisation Due to Falls by Older People (2005-2006) highlights these issues:

- The estimated number of hospitalised injury cases due to falls in people aged 65 years and over was 66,800.
- Older females accounted for most of the hospitalised fall injury cases and a third of cases had injuries to the hip and thigh.
- A fall on the same level, due to slipping, tripping and stumbling, was the most common cause of a hospitalised fall.
- Half of all fall injury cases for people aged 65 years and older occurred in the home.
- Older people who lived in aged care facilities were found to fall five times more than people of the same age who lived in the community and fell in their home.

Falls in New Zealand

The Injury Prevention Research Unit, Department of Preventive and Social Medicine, University of Otago, identified in February 2003 the 10 Leading Causes of Injury Resulting in Hospitalisations for New Zealand in 2000. In all 12 age categories the number one cause for hospital admission was falls. From 55 years of age onwards the percentage of people admitted as a result of a fall rose dramatically as follows:

- 55-64 years 41.6%
- 65-74years 60.5%

- 75-84 years 78%
- 85+ years 86.8%*

[* www.otago.ac.nz/ipru]

Risk factors for falls and fall-related injury included increasing age, a history of falls, limitation of activities of daily living, impaired cognition, a history of stroke or Parkinson's disease, psychoactive medication use and the use of more than four medications. Additional strong predictors of falls included impaired gait and mobility, impaired ability to stand, impaired ability with transfers, visual contrast sensitivity, decreased depth perception, reduced peripheral sensation, muscle weakness and poor reaction time.

Preventative strategies and responses

Falls often result in injury to older people but may also impact on their quality of life in a pervasive way. After a fall, older people may feel less confident and may impose restrictions on their own activities to avoid further incidents. It is therefore vitally important to consider how falls can be prevented in order to provide peace of mind for those at risk, as well as family members.

The goal of care is to prevent falls and fractures while at the same time preserve autonomy and promoting independence. The following is an extract of a Cochrane review (Gillespie et al., 2009) which evaluated successful interventions in a community cohort. This review examined which methods were effective in preventing falls in older people living in the community, and included a review of 111 randomised controlled trials, with a total of 55,303 participants. It concluded that:

- Exercise programs should target strength, balance, flexibility, and endurance. Programs that contain two or more of these components reduce the rate of falls and number of people falling. Exercising in supervised groups, participating in Tai Chi, and carrying out individually prescribed exercise programs at home are also effective.
- Some medications increase the risk of falling. Ensuring that medications are reviewed and adjusted may be effective in reducing falls. Gradual withdrawal from some types of drugs for improving sleep, reducing anxiety and treating depression has been shown to reduce falls.
- Cataract surgery reduces falls in people having the operation on the first affected eye. Insertion of a pacemaker can reduce falls in people with frequent falls associated with carotid sinus hypersensitivity, a condition which may result in changes in heart rate and blood pressure.

These outcomes are further reaffirmed by the evidence from 121 randomised controlled trials (6,700 participants) which demonstrated that older people who engage in strength training exercises become stronger. They also improve their performance of simple activities such as walking, climbing steps, or standing up from a chair more quickly. The improvement in activities such as getting out of a chair or stair climbing is generally greater than walking speed. Moreover, strength training exercises also improved older people's physical abilities, including more complex daily activities such as bathing or preparing a meal (Liu et al. 2006).

The impact of exercise on wellbeing in older people is increasingly recognised. The benefits of regular exercise offer numerous physical and mental health benefits. Strength and resistance training not only provide a greater sense of mental and physical wellbeing and reduction in falls and injury, but also appear to contribute to:

- Improved muscle size and strength and bone density
- Improved gait and balance and mobility
- Improved functional independence
- Improved mood, morale, insomnia and self-efficacy
- Treatment of wasting conditions
- Improved metabolism and disease control (Singh, Clements, and Fiatorone, 1997)

Despite this increasingly clear understanding of the contributors to falls in older people, we continue to be challenged about how this will realistically translate into practice. Dr. Jacqui Close (2006) has suggested we need to ask ourselves:

- Are older adults who present to Emergency Departments routinely assessed for falls risk?
- Are the visually impaired routinely offered an Occupational Therapy (OT) home assessment?
- Is cataract extraction being accelerated?

- Are doctors actively getting people off CNS acting medications?
- Are strength and balance training programs expanding to meet older adults' need?
- Do specialist falls services exist?

As most of these questions would be answered in the negative, it would appear that there is still much work to do to eliminate falls in older people.

Osteoporosis

Osteoporosis is the thinning and weakening of the bone substance and it increases the risk of fracture and deformity (Osteoporosis Australia website, 2009). Fractures, after minimal trauma, are a hallmark of osteoporosis. They can reduce a person's ability to walk unassisted and may lead to loss of independence. Osteoporosis has no symptoms and people often do not know that they have it until a fracture occurs. The disease is more common in females than in males and is mostly limited to older people (A Picture of Osteoporosis in Australia, 2008).

About 50% of people with one fracture due to osteoporosis will have another. The risk of future fractures rises with each new fracture – the 'cascade effect'. The 'cascade effect' means that women who have suffered a fracture in their spinal column are over four times more likely to have another fracture within the next year, compared to women who have never had an osteoporotic fracture. People who have had two or more osteoporotic fractures are up to nine times more likely to have another fracture, rising to a risk 11 times greater for people who have had three or more fractures, compared to someone who has not had one (Osteoporosis Australia website, 2009).

Prevention of osteoporosis

There are a number of ways to reduce the risk of osteoporosis. Weight-bearing exercise done regularly may be the most important. The physical stress put on bones during this exercise stimulates bone formation and thus helps maintain or increase bone density. Usually, 30 minutes of weight-bearing exercise each day is recommended. However, this should only be undertaken after a careful assessment has been carried out (Sambrook, et al., 2002).

Additionally, consuming enough calcium and vitamin D helps maintain bone density. Older people should consume 1,200 to 1,500 milligrams (mg) of calcium every day. Vitamin D plays an important role in calcium absorption and in bone health. It is made through exposure to sunlight. While many people are able to obtain enough vitamin D naturally, studies show that vitamin D production decreases in the elderly and in people who are housebound. These individuals may require vitamin D supplementation to ensure a daily intake of between 400 to 800IU of vitamin D (Osteoporosis New Zealand 2009).

Arthritis

Arthritis, osteoporosis and other diseases of the joints and bones place a significant burden on both the individual and community, including disruptions to daily life, use of hospital and primary care services and lost productivity. Almost one in five older Australians with arthritis or a musculoskeletal condition is reported to have some disability (Older Australians at a Glance, 2007).

Arthritis is an umbrella term for a number of medical conditions that affect the musculoskeletal system, specifically joints where two or more bones meet. The signs and symptoms of arthritis-related problems may include pain, stiffness, inflammation and damage to joint cartilage and surrounding structures. This can result in joint weakness, instability and deformities that can interfere with the most basic activities of daily living (Arthritis Australia website, 2009).

Arthritis is the major cause of disability and chronic pain in Australia (Higgins, Madjar and Walton, 2004), with 3.85million Australians affected at a cost to our economy of more than $23.9 billion each year in medical care and indirect costs such as loss of earnings and lost production (Arthritis Foundation, 2009). The incidence of chronic pain amongst older adults in nursing homes in New Zealand is very high (Higgins, Madjar and Walton, 2004), making pain management a serious challenge for aged care facility staff. Clearly, this will impact on residents' quality of life and may even contribute to the development of challenging behaviours in this population. Challenges are associated with effectively assessing older residents' pain and evaluating the most effective pharmacological and non-pharmacological means to control their pain (Higgins et al., 2004).

The most common forms of arthritis in an ageing population are osteoarthritis and rheumatoid arthritis.

Osteoarthritis may affect any joint in the body, though the knees and hands are most commonly affected, followed by the spine, hips, ankles and shoulders. Elbows and wrists aren't usually affected. Usually between one and four separate joints are involved.

In osteoarthritis:

- the cartilage loses elasticity and may split with pieces of cartilage breaking off and floating around in the synovial fluid;
- the cartilage may break down, leaving the bone exposed and unprotected;
- the bone loses shape and thickens at the rims of the joint, producing bony spurs called osteophytes;
- the bone beneath the joint surfaces often thins out;
- the muscles around the joint may waste away (Fact sheet – Osteoarthritis, Arthritis Australia website, 2009).

As these things happen, the joint loses its smooth functioning, becoming stiff and painful. In advanced stages of osteoarthritis the joint may be destroyed altogether and/or become dislocated (Merck Manual, 2004).

Osteoarthritis is more common in people who have a history of:

- continual stress on joints;
- weight problem;
- previous injury or surgery in a joint, especially if the joint didn't heal well;
- a genetic predisposition (ABS Health and Wellbeing website, 2009).

There is no cure for osteoarthritis but a variety of treatments can help people control and reduce the effects of the disease. Treatment aims to reduce pain and lessen stiffness as much as possible in order to improve joint function and mobility and to preserve quality of life as much as possible. This will most likely be achieved by the use the following strategies:

- use of analgesics and anti-inflammatory drugs to control pain and minimise inflammation;
- exercise to decrease pain, assist joint mobility, increase muscle strength, strengthen bones and ligaments, prevent joint deformities and increase fitness and general wellbeing. Gentle exercise is best, such as walking, Tai Chi and hydrotherapy;
- surgical treatments (in advanced situations) such as replacement of hips, knees and (less commonly) shoulders with artificial prostheses will relieve pain and improve mobility;
- keeping weight down means there is less stress on the hips and knees;

- minimising stresses on joints is achieved by being aware of activities and body positions that stress individual joints and aggravate the symptoms; and
- alternative treatments, two of the most common of which are glucosamine and chondroitin. These are dietary supplements that are also produced naturally in the body to make cartilage (Arthritis Australia, 2009).

Rheumatoid Arthritis (RA)

Rheumatoid arthritis is the most common autoimmune disease in Australia. RA causes pain, inflammation and swelling of the joints, leading to subsequent damage of joints. It usually affects smaller joints, such as those in the hands and feet, however, larger joints such as the hips and knees can also be affected.

The symptoms of RA vary from person to person although the most common symptoms are joint pain, swelling, tenderness to the touch and stiffness in the joints, especially in the mornings. RA is generally symmetrical with the same joints on both sides of the body being affected (McNeil, MEA, 2005).

Currently there is no cure for RA. However, treatments have improved dramatically over the past decade. Treatments will generally be tailored to an individual to meet the needs of the client and is dependent upon the severity of signs and symptoms of the condition.

Medicines that may be administered include non-steroidal anti-inflammatory drugs, corticosteroid medicines or injections, disease-modifying anti-rheumatic drugs and biological disease-modifying anti-rheumatic drugs, such as tumour necrosis factor medicines (Arthritis Australia website, 2009).

Issues of continence/incontinence

Incontinence has long evaded a widely accepted definition. Most definitions of urinary and faecal (or anal) incontinence describe a loss of control of urination or defecation respectively (AIHW, 2006, page 4).

Incontinence has been described as the accidental or involuntary loss of urine from the bladder (urinary incontinence) or bowel motion, faeces or wind from the bowel (faecal or bowel incontinence) (Continence Foundation of Australia (CFA), 2009).

Incontinence is a significant health issue across the lifespan, with physical, social and economic implications for the older person, their carers and the community. Almost four million Australians are estimated to have some level of incontinence, its prevalence increasing with age in both men and women (AIHW, 2006).

Urinary incontinence is a term used to describe losing control of your bladder. As a result, clothing may become damp or soaked. Incontinence relates to poor or lack of control and includes symptoms such as urgency and frequency.

Caregivers often identify incontinence as a significant contributing factor for moving a loved one into a long-term residential care facility, because of the substantial burden it places upon them.

It is believed that between 32-78% of older people in residential care experience urinary incontinence and between 10-72% experience faecal incontinence (AIHW, 2006).

Urinary incontinence is generally described as being of **four different types:**

Stress incontinence is involuntary leakage of urine during activities that increase pressure inside the abdomen, such as coughing, sneezing or jogging. Some older people with severe stress incontinence have nearly constant urine loss. This condition usually occurs because the urinary sphincter does not close adequately (CFA, 2009).

Urge incontinence (UI) is the inability to hold urine long enough to reach a toilet. It may occur as a result of a stroke or other central nervous system event, bladder infection or bladder tumour. UI is the most common type of persistent incontinence in older people. The cause of bladder overactivity and urge incontinence is usually unknown. Stroke, dementia or other disorders that affect the ability of the brain or spinal cord to inhibit bladder contractions when there is no opportunity to urinate may contribute. Additionally, conditions that irritate the bladder, such as atrophic vaginitis in women, prostate enlargement in men or severe constipation can also contribute to urge incontinence (New Zealand Continence Association website, 2009).

Overflow incontinence refers to a small continuous leak of urine associated with an overfull bladder that does not empty properly. This may occur because of an obstruction to the bladder or damage to the nerve supply. In older men, an enlarged prostate can block the urethra. Less commonly, scar tissue narrows or sometimes even blocks the lowest part of the bladder, where it connects to the urethra or blocks the urethra itself (urethral stricture). Such narrowing or blockage may occur after prostate surgery. Severe constipation or stool impaction can cause overflow incontinence if stools fills the rectum to the point of putting pressure on the lower portion of the bladder, the urinary sphincter or the urethra. Nerve damage that paralyses the bladder (a condition commonly called neurogenic bladder) can also cause overflow incontinence. Stroke and diabetes mellitus can paralyse the bladder, leading to overflow incontinence (CFA, 2009).

Functional incontinence is the difficulty reaching a toilet in time because of physical, mental or environmental conditions. The most common causes are conditions that lead to immobility, such as stroke or severe arthritis, and conditions that interfere with mental function, such as dementia. In rare cases, people become so depressed that they do not go to the toilet (known as psychogenic incontinence) (Merck Manual, 2004).

A thorough assessment of incontinence is necessary to determine its cause and characteristics. Additionally, the assessment process is structured to enable the clinician to detect any related system pathology, evaluate the patient comprehensively in relation to their mental and physical health, explore their history of medications and to investigate issues around their environment as well as determining the impact of the problem on their quality of life.

Managing urinary incontinence

Strategies for managing urinary incontinence are influenced largely by the cause of the incontinence. They should evolve around the assessment process and be individually tailored to the needs of the client within their environmental setting. In many cases, incontinence can be cured or reduced considerably. There is a range of interventions available and sometimes treatment may only involve education and some simple behavioural changes. Much will be dependent on the client's capacity to participate in any interventions or programs.

Strategies may evolve around pelvic floor muscle exercise to regain pelvic floor strength in those with stress incontinence to bladder training programs for those with urge incontinence and may additionally include surgical interventions and medications for those with overflow and functional incontinences.

Environmental issues to be addressed may include ensuring that the older person can actually find their way to the toilet, navigate obstacles appropriately, undo the necessary clothing and actually get to the toilet, in what is often a small amount of time from thought to desire to need.

Strategies may also be implemented which incorporate relevant responses to the review of medication (particularly diuretics and sedatives and tranquilizers) and fluid intakes, as well as assessment of mental health status (including mood).

Even those who are recognised as having urinary incontinence which will not respond to strategies and treatments can be additionally assisted with the use of more dignified and assistive aids and technologies (CFA, 2009; AIWI, 2006).

Faecal incontinence

Faecal (bowel) incontinence is the involuntary passing of faeces and/or flatus (wind) at an inappropriate time or place. It affects approximately 1% of people living in the community. It is a very distressing symptom and can affect a person physically, emotionally, socially and financially. Faecal incontinence is a symptom, not a disease, therefore it must be investigated to identify the cause (New Zealand Continence Association, 2009).

Poor bowel control is caused predominantly by diarrhoea or constipation but may also be a consequence of poor mobility, nerve injury or disease or damaged sphincter muscles around the back passage. Many people with poor bowel control will also have poor bladder control (AIHW, 2006).

Constipation

A normal bowel movement varies considerably from one person to another. Normal movement varies from three times a day to every three days. Importantly, your bowel is healthy if your bowel motions are: regular, soft and well formed, easy to pass and leave you feeling that your bowel has been fully emptied.

Constipation is a symptom, not a disease. It can be defined as a change from a normal bowel habit which can cause pain or discomfort. The bowel motion may be hard, dry and/or more difficult to pass. Contributing factors in older people may include:

- Decreased peristalsis due to age-related changes;
- Insufficient fluid intake (older people may restrict their fluid intake intentionally to (incorrectly) minimise urinary incontinence;
- Inadequate dietary fibre – it may also be a consequence of other nutritional issues;
- Ignoring the call to pass a motion;
- Poor seating position when moving your bowels;
- Lack of exercise and/or decreased mobility;
- Medical conditions and/or chronic illness;

- Medications (particularly opioids, analgesics, anti-cholinergics and anti-depressants);
- Long-term laxative use and abuse;
- Weakness, frailty and immobility;
- Anxiety, depression and grief;
- Various disorders of the bowel including malignancy; and
- Environmental factors (e.g. communal living and reduced privacy) (Wallis, 2003; Wilson, 2005; Merck Manual, 2004; Bladder and Bowel Website, 2009; CFA, 2009)

Managing constipation

The Joanna Briggs institute provides an evidence-based information sheet on constipation and its management which provides the following summary of recommendations for management*:

[* http://www.joannabriggs.edu.au/pdf/BP_Book_Vol12_7.pdf]

Prevention is better than cure so it is recommended that older adults receive advice and education about hydration and a good diet with fibre sources, including cereals, nuts and seeds, whole meal breads, cooked and raw vegetables and fruits;

Older adult patients require screening for history of medication use (especially polypharmacy and taking of laxatives) and cognitive status;

- For persons unable to walk or who are restricted to bed or otherwise incapacitated, exercises such as low trunk rotation and pelvic tilt are advised;

- Monitoring and recording of bowel movements for frequency, character, pattern, episodes of constipation/faecal spoiling and use of oral or rectal laxative; and
- Osmotic laxatives such as PEG and lactulose and bulking agents like psyllium and bran are beneficial in managing constipation in older adults and should be promoted; it is necessary to determine individual requirements.

Diarrhoea

Diarrhoea is the passing of frequent, urgent loose bowel motions and has many possible causes including:

- the use of stimulant laxatives, especially if overused or used incorrectly;
- bowel or stomach infection;
- bowel diseases;
- specific medications (e.g. antibiotics);
- a shortened bowel (following surgery to remove some of the bowel);
- food allergies and food intolerance;
- alcohol;
- radiotherapy; and
- impacted faeces – with an overflow which may present and/or be reported as diarrhoea.

Diarrhoea requires investigation to identify the cause, followed by implementation of appropriate strategies. Diarrhoea can be more difficult to control than formed motions and older people may require additional support to assist them through this experience.

A part of good aged care is for nursing staff to be mindful about the continence needs of older clients. Regular observation and investigation is required to document these accurately and to take a preventative approach to these issues.

Faecal incontinence that does not respond to treatment and strategies is a very distressing problem for the client and family and the overriding aim of care is to maintain dignity and demonstrate respect through the use of appropriate aids, appliances and resources.

Ultimately the identification of urinary or faecal incontinence alters significantly the care of an older person and may contribute to a loss of self-esteem and cause social isolation and depression, particularly for those older people who have insight into these problems.

It should never be accepted as an inevitable outcome of ageing (even in those with advanced cognitive decline) and the emphasis of care should always be to maintain continence for all older people.

Diabetes

Diabetes is categorised as type 1 or type 2, each having a different cause. The most common type of diabetes among older people is type 2 diabetes. Diabetes is extremely common in older people, of whom about 15-25% have the disease. Obese older people with a family history of diabetes have the highest risk of developing type 2 diabetes in which the body does not respond normally to the insulin produced, or the body may not make enough insulin (Diabetes Australia website, 2009).

Diagnosis and treatment of diabetes in older people is often complicated by the presence of age-related changes and comorbidities. When diabetes is under-treated or poorly managed, older people are more likely to experience greater morbidity, disability and death as a result (Dunning, T 2005).

Diabetes accounted for 13% of hospital separations in the over 65 year old age group in 2004–05, according to Australian hospital data. For this cohort, 47% of hospital separations were for eye complications (ophthalmic), 13% for multiple complications, 12% for other specified complications of diabetes, 9% for circulatory complications, 8% for renal complications and 7% for poor control (Diabetes Australia, 2009).

Long-term complications include disease of large blood vessels, leading to conditions such as coronary heart disease, stroke and peripheral vascular disease, and disease of small blood vessels, causing chronic kidney disease, nerve damage and retinopathy (loss of vision) (Older Australians at a Glance, 2007).

Often symptoms of diabetes go unnoticed as the disease develops. Symptoms may include blurred vision, skin infections, slow healing, tingling and numbness in the feet. Sometimes no symptoms are noticed at all. A fasting blood sugar level is most commonly used to make the diagnosis (Merck Manual, 2004).

Occasionally, blood glucose levels in people with type 2 diabetes become extremely high. Extremely high levels often result from failing to take drugs to control blood sugar or from stress to the body, such as infection or surgery.

Once diabetes has been diagnosed, the person should be screened for disease complications at least once a year. This should include examination of the person's feet for any signs of poor blood flow, decreased sensation, skin breakdown and infection.

Treatments for diabetics are individually tailored with the goal of maintaining blood glucose levels within the normal range in order to prevent or control symptoms and reduce the risk of developing complications. Treatment involves a range of options and includes diet, exercise, drugs and frequent monitoring of blood glucose levels, all of which are underpinned by education for the client and those supporting them.

The dietary approach to diabetes management has undergone numerous changes in recent years. The traditional 'diabetic diet' gives little benefit for blood glucose control and may place individuals at nutritional risk. It is now recognised that moderate amounts of sugar can be included in the diets of people with diabetes. The emphasis is on selecting a variety of nutritious foods, based on high fibre, carbohydrates and a low intake of saturated fats. A good balance of foods can improve blood glucose management, general wellbeing and assist with weight maintenance (Diabetes Australia, 2009).

Dietary measures alone are sometimes enough to maintain a healthy weight and control blood sugar levels. People with diabetes should be physically active. Putting extra physical activity into ordinary activities, such as walking instead of driving to a store or taking stairs instead of elevators, can often help. However, formal exercise is often needed.

Drug therapy is started when diet and exercise do not adequately lower blood sugar levels or when a person's living conditions, physical strength or motivation make proper diet and exercise impossible.

Oral anti-hyperglycaemic drugs are usually the first drugs given. Insulin is required if anti-hyperglycaemic drugs alone cannot control blood sugar levels adequately. Temporary insulin treatment is also sometimes necessary during periods of high physical stress. Insulin is divided into four basic types based on how quickly it works and how long it lasts.

It is essential for people with diabetes to regularly monitor their blood glucose levels. Some people check their blood glucose only once or twice a day, whilst others check it more than 4 times a day. Most blood sugar monitoring devices use only a tiny drop of blood which is obtained by pricking the tip of the finger with a small lancet. It may be necessary to undertake this role on behalf of a client who is cognitively impaired or physically unable to undertake this task.

The most common complication of treating high blood glucose levels is low blood glucose levels. Common symptoms of low blood glucose include sweating, nausea, warmth, anxiety, shakiness, palpitations, hunger, headache, blurred or double vision, confusion and difficulty speaking. In the worst cases, low blood glucose can cause coma, permanent brain damage and even death. For this reason, low blood glucose levels must be treated immediately (Diabetes New Zealand, 2009).

A short-acting form of glucose must be introduced into the body within minutes to relieve symptoms of low blood glucose and prevent harm to the brain. When glucose is unavailable or the person is unconscious, emergency medical personnel may have to inject glucose into a vein.

Despite being an increasingly common occurrence in ageing, diabetes is manageable if education and treatments are provided as part of a sound holistic plan.

Cardiovascular disease

Cardiovascular disease is an embracing term which refers to all diseases and conditions of the heart and blood vessels. The main underlying cause of cardiovascular disease is atherosclerosis, a process marked by abnormal build-ups of fat, cholesterol and other substances in the inner lining of the arteries. It is most serious when it reduces or blocks blood supply to the heart (causing angina or heart attack) or to the brain (causing a stroke).

Cardiovascular problems in older age may affect quality of life, length of life or both. Of these diseases, coronary heart disease (CHD), stroke, heart failure and peripheral vascular disease (PVD) are major contributors to the disease burden in Australia and have their greatest impact among older Australians. The 'burden of disease' is a measure of the amount of ill health, disability and premature death caused by individual disease or health conditions (Older Australians at a Glance, p.63).

Coronary heart disease (CHD)

This is almost always caused by atherosclerosis. In atherosclerosis, cholesterol and other materials are deposited in the wall of an artery, forming plaques. As these plaques enlarge, they partially or completely block the artery. Occasionally, a blood clot forms on a plaque, making the degree of blockage greater and sometimes blocking the artery completely.

CHD, also known as ischaemic heart disease, is the most common form of heart disease. There are two major clinical forms; heart attack (often known as acute myocardial infarction or AMI) and angina (Older Australians at a Glance, 2007).

A myocardial infarction (heart attack) is a life-threatening event that occurs when a blood vessel supplying the heart itself is suddenly blocked completely, threatening to damage the heart and its functions. An angina attack is a temporary chest pain or discomfort that occurs when the heart's own blood supply is inadequate to meet extra needs, such as during exercise (National Heart Foundation website, 2009).

Angina

Angina is a symptom of myocardial ischaemia. Complaints of vague discomfort under the sternum may be one of the first symptoms especially after exercise or a meal. Angina is often described as pressure, tightness, squeezing or heaviness (like a weight on the chest). It may be felt only in the chest, or it may move. Most commonly, it moves down the left arm. It may move to the back, throat, neck, jaw, teeth or right arm. The discomfort usually develops gradually and subsides gradually after a few minutes (up to about 20 minutes). Angina is usually relieved by resting or by taking nitroglycerin, placed or sprayed under the tongue. Occasionally, angina is accompanied by shortness of breath, nausea, dizziness or fatigue. Older people may also break out in a cold sweat or have palpitations. In some people, the only symptom may be shortness of breath that is triggered by physical activity or stress (Merck Manual, 2004; National Heart Foundation, 2009).

Several different types of drugs may be prescribed to treat stable angina. If drugs are not effective or if the blockage is substantial, angioplasty or coronary artery bypass graft surgery may be necessary. Both procedures are good options for older people and both relieve symptoms and may prolong life. Which procedure is done depends largely on the location and degree of the blockage (Rawlings-Anderson, et al., 2003; RACGP Guidelines, Coronary Syndromes, 2006)

Myocardial infarction

Symptoms of a myocardial infarction are similar to those of myocardial ischemia, but they usually last longer and are more severe. As with angina, pain due to a heart attack may be felt in the chest, neck, throat, jaw, teeth or arms. However, in older people, a heart attack may cause little or no chest pain or discomfort. Instead, a heart attack may cause shortness of breath, a smothering feeling, nausea, vomiting, sweating, dizziness, indigestion, palpitations, overwhelming fatigue, fainting, a feeling of impending doom or any combination of these symptoms. Less commonly, older people who are having a heart attack become confused, disoriented, or restless. About one quarter of all heart attacks occur without symptoms, as silent heart attacks (Merck Manual, 2004).

Getting emergency treatment as soon as possible can reduce the amount of damage done to the heart and increase the chances of a good recovery. The main goals of treatment are to improve blood flow through the coronary arteries, relieve symptoms and prevent additional problems.

Anyone with angina that is worsening (unstable angina) or with symptoms that may indicate a heart attack should take one aspirin, call an emergency telephone number and get to a hospital immediately (if not already in hospital). The aspirin should be chewed so that it is absorbed more quickly (National Heart Foundation website, 2009).

While treatment is being started, electrocardiography and blood tests are done. If these tests confirm unstable angina or a heart attack, additional treatments may be given including anti-platelet drugs that help prevent new blood clots from forming in the coronary artery (Acute Coronary Care Guidelines, 2006).

Coronary angiography (cardiac catheterisation) is the most accurate way to detect CHD and to determine the extent and location of blockages. This information helps doctors decide which treatments are best and whether angioplasty or bypass surgery is needed (National Heart Foundation, 2009).

Additional treatments may be needed for problems that develop after a heart attack, such as abnormal heart rhythms, heart failure or pulmonary oedema. Sometimes computed tomography (CT Coronary Angiography) is used to detect CHD, confirm the diagnosis or check for calcium that can accumulate in plaques in coronary arteries. This test is simple, safe, quick and painless.

Coronary angioplasty is used to physically open a blocked coronary artery. This procedure is often preferred to bypass surgery because it is less invasive. However, angioplasty may be impossible because the affected area is too large or there are too many blockages to be treated effectively with angioplasty (Brown and Edwards, 2005). A thin catheter with a balloon at its tip is threaded into the blocked coronary artery. Inflating the balloon opens up the artery. Often, a small tube made of wire mesh (stent) is inserted at the same time. Angioplasty with a stent is more likely to prevent the artery from becoming blocked again than is angioplasty alone (National Heart Foundation, 2009).

In coronary artery bypass graft surgery (commonly called bypass surgery) a vein or an artery from another part of the body is used to bypass the blocked coronary artery. Bypass surgery is usually recommended when there are several blockages or when the blockages occur throughout the length of a coronary artery. In such cases, angioplasty is unlikely to be effective. More than half of people who have bypass surgery are aged 65 or over (Merck Manual 2004).

Bypass surgery is routine and relatively safe. However, risks are higher for older people than for younger ones, partly because older people are more likely to have other disorders that increase risk (such as diabetes, lung disorders or kidney disorders). Problems that can occur after bypass surgery include strokes, abnormal heart rhythms, temporary confusion, difficulty breathing, pulmonary embolism, bleeding, infections, kidney failure and death (National Heart Foundation, 2009).

Prevention of CAD revolves around eliminating modifiable risk factors. This means that a focus on stopping smoking (the benefit of stopping smoking is at least as great for older people as for younger people), controlling or lowering blood pressure and cholesterol and weight reducing diets with regular exercise will impact significantly on the incidence of CAD (Brown and Edwards et al., 2005).

Stroke

Stroke occurs when the supply of blood to the brain is suddenly disrupted. Blood may stop moving through an artery because the artery is blocked by a blood clot or plaque (ischaemic stroke), or because the artery breaks or bursts (haemorrhagic stroke). Strokes are Australia's second single greatest killer after coronary heart disease and a leading cause of disability in older people (National Stroke Foundation website, 2009).

Common stroke symptoms are the sudden onset of loss of strength or feeling of the face, arm and/or leg on one side of the body, loss of normal speech, loss of balance and loss of normal vision (Merck Manual, 2004).

A number of tests may be done in hospital to confirm the diagnosis of stroke, including a CT scan or MRI to determine the type of stroke and the part of the brain affected.

When the signs of stroke are present but go away within 24 hours, the term Transient Ischaemic Attack (TIA) is used. The causes and symptoms of a TIA are similar to those of a stroke.

TIA episodes usually last a few minutes to a few hours. They generally disappear quickly and are often ignored because of their brevity. About one in five people who have a TIA will have a major stroke within the next three months and a large part of the risk occurs in the first few days. Therefore, TIAs should never be ignored and, just like a stroke, will require emergency treatment (National Stroke Foundation, 2009).

The main risk factors for stroke are:

- high blood pressure;
- cigarette smoking;
- high blood cholesterol;
- diabetes;
- heavy alcohol use and 'binge' drinking;
- existing heart and blood vessel disease, including disorders of heart rhythm (such as atrial fibrillation), coronary heart disease and peripheral arterial disease;
- previous stroke or transient ischaemic attack (TIA); and
- increasing age.

(National Heart Foundation, 2009)

Therefore, reducing the risk of stroke requires the recognising and controlling of hypertension, cessation of smoking, monitoring and treating cholesterol levels, maintaining healthy non-fat diets, reducing or ceasing alcohol consumption, maintaining regular physical activity and, if in a high risk category, regular use of a blood thinning agent. Surgery may also be used to remove fatty deposits, particularly in the carotids, if this is supported by investigation and diagnosis (RACGP Guidelines, 2008).

Following a stroke it is clear that the best outcomes for older people are achieved by those who are cared for in a specialised stroke unit followed by a significant stay in a rehabilitation unit (National Stroke Foundation, 2009).

Visual deficits

About 170,000 Australians aged 65 years and over have visual impairment caused by eye disease. Of these, 51,000 people are classified as blind and almost 119,000 others have low vision. There is a strong association between visual impairment and advancing age (Older Australians at a Glance, 2007).

Visual impairment can affect physical, functional, emotional and social wellbeing and markedly reduce quality of life. The ability to perform basic activities of daily living can be affected, leading to less independence. Visual deficits are also a significant contributor to falls in the elderly (Lord, et al., 2005).

Presbyopia

Presbyopia is the condition in which the natural lens of the eye loses its flexibility so that focusing on close objects becomes difficult. It is viewed as part of normal ageing and is treated with the use of prescription glasses which require ongoing assessment and evaluation.

Additional significant causes of visual impairment in the older generation which are not considered normal are cataracts, agerelated macular degeneration and glaucoma.

Cataracts

Cataracts are the most common eye disease among Australians aged 65 and over, affecting over 1.2 million people. Age-specific rates for cataract increase with age and are well over 70% for people aged 80 years and over. Generally, prevalence rates are higher among women than among men (Older Australians at a Glance, 2007).

Cataracts create a clouding of the lens or capsule of the eye and cause the lens to become less transparent. Visual acuity becomes progressively distorted and night vision decreased and objects may become blurred. Glare becomes uncomfortable. Surgical intervention includes removing the lens and replacement it with an intraocular lens (Centre for Eye Research, 2009).

Age-related macular degeneration (AMD)

This is the leading cause of blindness among Australians aged 65 years and over. AMD is a progressive condition which involves damage to the macular of the retina that provides fine vision for daily tasks such as reading and recognising faces. Laser treatment may be used for some causes of macular degeneration (as a result of infection or injury), however, it is often not as successful for the age-related type (Macular Degeneration Foundation website, 2009).

Glaucoma

This degenerative disease involves damage to the optic nerve and subsequent vision loss or blindness from increased intraocular pressure. It is a major cause of blindness and increases in prevalence with age.

In acute glaucoma (closed-angle) the older person experiences severe eye pain, headaches and gastro-intestinal upset. Vision becomes blurred and blindness will result if it is not corrected (Mitchell, et al., 2005).

The chronic form (open-angle) is more common and more gradual in its development. Peripheral vision becomes gradually and progressively affected and central vision is eventually affected.

Tunnel vision may develop and only objects that are straight ahead of the person can be seen. Eyes may feel tired, vision may be misty or the person may see halos around objects, and the individual may complain of headaches. The cornea may look cloudy and the iris fixed and dilated (Glaucoma Australia Inc., 2009).

Although there is no cure for glaucoma it can usually be controlled and further loss of sight either prevented or at least slowed down.

Treatments include various eye drops to suit the patient and the glaucoma, laser treatment or surgery where a new channel is created for fluid to leave the eye (Eye Foundation, 2009).

Hearing loss

Among the older population approximately a third has significant hearing loss by age 65 and one half of the cohort by age 80. Hearing loss can have a profound effect on quality of life, especially when it interferes with the ability to hear and understand speech (Smith et al., 2005; Hogan et al., 2009).

Hearing loss due to ageing usually develops gradually. Highpitched sounds are affected more than low-pitched sounds. An inability to hear the sounds of some consonants may make it sound as if a speaker is mumbling (Merck Manual, 2004).

Conversations become difficult to follow, particularly in crowded or noisy areas. Constantly asking others to talk louder can frustrate both the listener and the speaker. People with hearing loss may misunderstand a question and give an apparently distorted or inappropriate response, leading others to believe they are confused.

Hearing aid manufacturers purport to improve quality of life for the majority of older people with hearing loss but many older people would disagree with that proposition. Many older people have great difficulty adjusting to the sound differences with hearing aids and, because of these difficulties and often a lack of support from professionals and family, discard them claiming to hear better without them (Proceedings MACA, 2003).

One of the important barriers to coping with hearing loss is overcoming the embarrassment that some older people experience related to wearing a hearing aid. Many people in the community see this as an opportunity to reinforce ageist stereotypes and treat older people with hearing aids as if they have advanced cognitive impairment rather than a hearing impairment. This is another contributing factor to older people often choosing not to wear their hearing aids.

Those people who cannot benefit from hearing aids may be helped by a cochlear implant which is becoming increasingly performed on older clients.

Respect, kindness, patience and time are required to communicate effectively with someone who has a hearing loss. One would hope that even in our fast paced and busy world these are essential qualities within our aged care workforce.

Common cancers of ageing

Prostate cancer

Prostate cancer is the most commonly registered cancer in older males, followed by colorectal cancer, lung cancer and melanoma (Older Australians at a Glance 2007).

Each year in Australia, close to 3,000 men die of prostate cancer and around 18,700 new cases are diagnosed in Australian every year.

Prostate cancer can be cured if detected and treated while still confined to the prostate gland (Prostate Cancer Foundation, 2009).

The tests for prostate cancer are the prostate specific antigen (PSA) blood test and the digital rectal examination (DRE). These tests do not give a conclusive diagnosis of cancer but can indicate the presence of prostate cancer. Symptoms may include one or more of the following:

- Waking frequently at night to urinate;
- Sudden or urgent need to urinate;
- Difficulty in starting to urinate;
- Slow flow of urine and difficulty in stopping;
- Discomfort when urinating;
- Painful ejaculation;
- Blood in the urine or semen;
- Decrease in libido; and

- Reduced ability to get an erection.

(Prostate Cancer Foundation, 2009)

Prostate cancer treatments continue to advance and the response is always a personalised one based on the informed needs and desires of the client. Additionally, preferences are influenced by the age and condition of the client and the history and infiltration of the cancer.

Treatments range from doing nothing to undertaking an active surveillance/watchful waiting approach to surgical interventions and/or various types of guided radiotherapies, prostate seed brachytherapy, hormone therapy and high intensity focused Ultrasound (Prostate Cancer Foundation of Australia, 2009)

Breast cancer

In older females, breast cancer is the most commonly registered cancer, followed by colorectal cancer, lung cancer and melanoma. Breast cancer is the leading cause of death in older females and the single largest risk for developing cancer is age (Older Australians at a Glance, 2007).

Less than 1% of all people diagnosed with breast cancer are men. Breast cancer in men is, however, on the rise with about 100 men being diagnosed in Australia in 2008. Breast cancer develops in either the ducts or the lobules. Lobules are where the milk is produced and ducts are where the milk travels to the nipple. Cancer cells develop when the cells lining the ducts or lobules become abnormal in size and shape and start multiplying in an uncontrolled way (National Breast Cancer Foundation website, 2009).

It is not possible to say what exactly causes breast cancer. However, research has shown that some factors might increase a woman's risk or chance of developing breast cancer. The main risk factors for developing breast cancer appear to be:

- Being female;
- Having a strong family history of breast cancer, although the majority of people who are diagnosed have no known family history;
- Inheriting a faulty gene (a gene mutation) that increases the risk of breast cancer; and
- Having previously been diagnosed with breast cancer. (McGrath Foundation website, 2009)

Women over 50 years of age should be even more aware of breast cancer risk if they have other risk factors for breast cancer, including:

- Being Caucasian;
- Having had their first child after age 30;
- Having used hormone replacement therapy;
- Never having had children;
- Smoking cigarettes; and
- Started menopause after age 50.

(AIHW, National Breast and Ovarian Cancer Centre, 2009)

Changes to look for in a breast include:

- A lump or thickening in the breast or armpit;
- A change in the size or shape of your breast;
- Skin changes such as dimpling or redness;

- Nipple inversion or discharge;
- Change to the nipple, like a rash, ulcer or itchiness; and
- An unusual or persistent pain.

(National Breast Cancer Foundation, 2009)

These changes may prompt a clinical examination by a health professional, a mammogram or ultrasound or a fine needle or core biopsy which would contribute to a diagnosis being made.

Breast cancer may be diagnosed as contained within the milk ducts or milk sacs, within the breast with no spread, be diagnosed locally advanced to lymph nodes or other areas around the breast or be secondary or metastatic with spread to other organs and places within the body.

Treatment regimes for breast cancer are dependent on a number of factors and will vary according to these factors and the stage of the cancer. Each woman's situation is personalised as is each treatment regime. The primary aim of breast cancer treatment for all is to remove the breast cancer, destroy any cancer cells that may remain in the breast and surrounding area and to destroy any cancer cells that may have spread outside the breast.

Breast cancer treatment can include surgery, chemotherapy, radiotherapy and hormonal therapies. It may also include specific drugs for particular types of breast cancer.

Summary

In various aged care settings aged care nurses deliver 24 hour care to their older clients. Increasingly there is a need for this care to be underpinned by knowledge, understanding and appreciation of contemporary aged care issues. This chapter has contributed to a knowledge of older adults' common health problems by providing an overview of these and their treatment highlighting wellness and prevention approaches in aged care settings and the community.

Chapter 9

Mental health and illness in old age

Regina McDonald
Area Clinical Nurse Consultant, Specialist Mental Health Services for Older People, SSWAHS &

Brian McMinn, RN, MHN, BSc., MNurs (NP), FACMHN
Clinical Nurse Consultant, Mental Health of Older People,
Hunter New England Mental Health Service; Conjoint Lecturer,
Faculty of Health University of Newcastle

Objectives

This chapter will enable the reader to:

1) Define the role of the aged care psychiatry nurse;
2) Understand the social context in relation to the older person who is experiencing a mental health problem;
4) Describe some common mental health problems in old age;
5) Understand the need for comprehensive assessments for older adults with a mental health problem;

6) Explain the outcome measures and assessment tools used in aged care psychiatry;
7) Examine the reasons for using outcome measures in aged care psychiatry;
8) Discuss nursing interventions and management of mental illness in old age; and
9) Illustrate health promotion principles in relation to mental health problems in old age.

Introduction

The structure of the population of Australia and the rest of the world is changing, expanding and ageing. This has been described elsewhere in this book. As a result of the exponential growth of the elderly, particularly the very old (85 years and over), there is a need for health care professionals to learn more about determinants of health for this segment of the population and the impact this has on mental and physical health. The social and economic implications of this increase are yet to be truly witnessed as the largest cohort of the post-war period are now beginning to age and retire.

Good health is considered by older adults to be a crucial factor to successful ageing and includes psychological factors (such as adaptation and acceptance) and emotional wellbeing (Reichstadt, Depp, Palinkas, Folsom, and Jeste, 2007, p.195). Older people consider themselves to be in excellent, very good or good health although this changes with advancing age (Australian Government, 2008, p.293). However, not all older people will age well and many from this cohort could develop diseases and disorders whose incidence will increase with age (Ames and Ritchie, 2007, p.452) and may well include physical and cognitive decline. Additionally, some will potentially experience financial and social hardships which in turn may result in significant mental health problems.

Mental health nursing of older people

Older people with mental health problems are nursed in acute care, community health-related service settings, community-based care programs supporting them in their home and low and high care residential aged care facilities. The brief of the nurse caring for the older adult is to assist the older adult to maintain the greatest degree of functioning and optimal level of health and wellbeing that is possible, and to assist them to meet their physical, psychological, social and spiritual needs. The nurse must be able to recognise and acknowledge the intrinsic and extrinsic factors contributing to an older client's ill health. The psychogeriatric nurse (sometimes called Older Persons Mental Health Nurse) is expected to have advanced knowledge in gerontology, geriatrics and mental health, an understanding of the nursing process and skills and competence surrounding its implementation. Additionally, an appreciation of the social context in which mental illness may manifest and the management options available are also mandatory if effective and appropriate consumer and carer outcomes are to be achieved in contemporary mental health nursing of the older person.

Mental health in old age

Mental health is the ability to cope and feel positive about others and to manage events in one's life. This is unlike mental illness, which significantly interferes with one's thoughts, feelings or social behaviour (NSW Institute of Psychiatry, 2007, p.2).

Mental illness and disorders may result from a combination of factors, including physical ill health, and is often associated with adverse psychological and social factors. These causes may interfere with the older person's thought processes and emotional feelings, and may result in socially unacceptable behaviour. Mental illness may include mood disorders (for example, major depression and bipolar disorder), schizophrenia and some of the personality disorders (Hansson, 2006, p.46). The most common mental illness in older people is depression and the most common mental disorder is dementia, with behaviour and psychological symptoms of dementia more commonly referred to as BPSD.

Mental health in the social context

Consideration must be given to the duration of the illness and the impact of psychosocial functioning when assessing the severity of mental illness (Hansson, 2006), particularly in the older person. The medical model is inadequate for addressing issues related to assessment and management options for the older person. The social model, encompassing of the physical, psychological, social and environmental domains, is more appropriate in order to restore older people to their most optimal level of physical and mental functioning following a period of ill health. To maximise the capacity to achieve this, each person's limitations must be acknowledged and their remaining strengths acknowledged and reinforced. While physical disability, poor physical health and chronic pain may contribute to the development of mental health problems in older adults, social factors may also contribute significantly. These may include loss and grief, social isolation, declining roles and a fear of becoming a burden to family. Mental illness is not a consequence of ageing but is fast becoming a major public health issue (NSW Institute of Psychiatry, 2007, p.1) and the aged are not quarantined from the morbidity that is often a consequence of mental illness.

Mental health services in Australia and New Zealand

As Australia comprises six states and two territories, there is a lack of a cohesive policy for mental health service provision. Legal differences also are evident, with some states not viewing dementia as a mental illness. There is also a lack of adequate services provided by some states and territories whilst others have no plan for how to deal with behavioural and psychological symptoms associated with dementia. Funding of services, team structures and the number of acute psychogeriatric services is also variable between states and territories. Aged Care Assessment Teams (ACATs) provide assessment for older people with mental health problems, while aged care packages offer support and respite care in the community. The number of psychogeriatricians and psychogeriatric nurses also varies considerably across states and territories.

In New Zealand, 15 out of 21 District Health Boards provide dedicated psychogeriatric services. Multidisciplinary community assessment teams assess and treat older patients at home. Back up medical services are provided by hospitals. There is a great variability in the number of acute inpatient beds across the country. Long stay beds, respite and day care are provided in the private sector by private for-profit and not-for-profit organisations. There are few psychogeriatric day hospitals (Draper, Melding and Brodaty, 2007).

Depression

The presentation of depression in old age is often less obvious than it is in younger people. Depression in the older person can often mimic dementia and may present with some of the same symptoms, for example, memory impairment, disordered judgement and alterations in general functioning. Many older people have at least one physical disability and depressed elderly patients are likely to focus attention on physical symptoms when dealing with health services or seeking help. Depression, therefore, can easily be overlooked in the elderly. Moreover, older adults may attribute their symptoms (lack of energy, inability to concentrate, irritability, poor sleep, weight loss and fatigue) to their age, rather than to a psychological cause.

The cardinal features of depression are lowered mood and loss of interest in the usual activities that they would normally be interested in when they are well. However, older people may be less likely than younger patients to acknowledge feeling depressed.

The term 'depression' does not necessarily result in a particular diagnosis. Non-typical, less obvious and less severe cases, especially those where there is co-morbidity with physical disorders, and where anxiety and certain personality traits can obscure the presentation, are not easily categorised under systems such as DSM-IV-TR (2005). It is relatively easy to recognise severe cases, but depression in non-melancholic cases, including what used to be called 'neurotic' or 'reactive' depression, is harder to recognise (Snowdon, 2001). Psychotic features of delusions and hallucinations can also be present in the depressed elderly.

Risk factors for depression

Risk factors for depression are multiple and complex and can be considered under physical, psychological, social and environmental domains. Psychological, social and environmental risks include losses and bereavement, previous episodes of major depression, previous sustained depressive responses to life events, pronounced dysfunctional personality traits (for example, obsessive, dependent), other psychiatric disorders, relocation to a new and different environment and being in a constant and difficult caring role (for example, caring for a spouse who has dementia or other chronic illness). Physical risks for mental health problems include chronic or potentially life-threatening physical illness, substance dependence and abuse and chronic pain. Some medications may cause or aggravate mood symptoms, including anti-hypertensives, steroids, analgesics, anti-Parkinson medications, anti-psychotics and benzodiazepines (Baldwin, Chiu, Katona and Graham, 2002).

Some presentations which may lead to the suspicion of depression include somatic and autonomic symptoms (pain, hypochondriasis) and poor concentration. Bodily or vegetative signs (including sleep disturbance, appetite change and reduced energy levels) are complaints that predict major depression and the requirement for treatment. Depressed mood, expressions of guilt and suicidal ideation occurring together are common depressive symptoms.

Nursing interventions

Below is a brief selection of helpful nursing interventions for older adults who are experiencing depression:

- **Supportive therapy** refers to the sustained engagement of the person focused on the understanding of symptoms and ventilation of problems.
- **Reminiscence therapy** involves a focus on positive life events.
- **Cognitive therapy** is about questioning or challenging distorted ways of thinking and illogical negative beliefs in an attempt to reduce pessimism, focusing on hope.
- **Problem solving** assists with clarifying choices faced by the person in day-to-day living.
- **Behaviour therapy** suggests that there be structured involvement in pleasurable events, avoidance of unpleasant activities and the monitoring of mood diaries. This includes involvement in exercise; progressive resistance training (Singh, Clements and Fiatarone, 1997) and encouragement to renew social contacts.
- **Interpersonal therapy** refers to strategies to improve important relationships in the person's life.
- **Support of psychiatric treatments** includes administering medications, information giving, moni-

toring the older person's progress and assistance with and interpretation of diagnostic tests.

- **Assistance with self-care and instrumental ADLs** includes re-motivating the older person to carry out self-care activities through graded withdrawal of assistance.
- **Maintenance of nutrition and hydration** is particularly important, especially if reduced appetite and significant weight loss is present.
- **Environment change** includes encouraging change to where light, good ventilation and sensory stimulation are present.

Treatment and management options for depression

Depression requires a psychosocial model for assessment and treatment and a community focus of ongoing management and care. Most depressive episodes in old age will respond to treatment, with a subsequent improvement in physical functioning and feelings of wellbeing, an improvement in physical and medical health status and reduced mortality. Improvement may occur with treatment, but early relapse and treatment resistance are common. Co-morbid physical disorders or severe anxiety may also lead to a protracted course. Overall, the prognosis for late-life depression is no worse than for younger patients. Older adults may take longer to respond, and treatment is often complicated, but there is good reason to be positive (Anderson, 2001; Snowdon, 2001).

If assessment reveals an obvious cause for the depression it should be appropriately treated. For example, relevant physical disorders should be identified and treated. Situations or drugs which are contributing to the depression should be changed if feasible. If the person is suicidal or has severe or psychotic depression, referral to specialist services is advisable and inpatient admission or specialist community care should be considered. Other issues indicating a need for specialist input are threats to safety of self or others through disturbed behaviour, new or significant cognitive deterioration, association with new physical illness and/or treatment (for example, medications), diagnostic uncertainty and treatment failure.

Electroconvulsive Therapy

Electroconvulsive Therapy (ECT) is considered to be as effective if not superior to pharmacological treatments in severe depression (van der Wurff, 2003; Heffern, 2000). However, relapse is frequent, often requiring maintenance ECT and/or anti-depressants. Indications include life-threatening situations due to suicidal behaviour or food refusal, anti-depressant treatment resistance, past history of response and medical conditions precluding antidepressants use (for example, renal, cardiac or hepatic conditions).

Suicide

Suicide is a tragedy no matter which age group is affected. Rates of suicide for older men are about as high as that for younger men and rates for older women are about the same as the general population.

Suicide in older people is characterised by few warnings or cues, high lethality due to frailty or intent to die, little history of previous attempts, greater prevalence of depression in the context of physical illness, hopelessness and less likelihood of contacting mental health services. Older people may not disclose their feelings because of the shame related to having mental health problems or fear about the consequences. A significant proportion of people who die by suicide have seen their health care provider in the three months prior to death (however, the visit may not be specifically about suicidal ideation). Older people do not generally access mental health services, receiving their health care from doctors, community centres and hospitals. Elderly suicide attempters remain both physically and mentally vulnerable after the suicide attempt. A repeat act represents a turning point in the older person's life progression and is essential to detect (Lebret et al., 2006).

Risk factors for suicide

Suicide risk can be assessed by considering 'risk' and 'resilience factors'. Suicide risk is variable and cannot be assessed during only one interview. The overall aim of suicide prevention is to help older people recognise their strengths and assist them in finding solutions to their problems.

Risk factors (escalating in severity) include:

- age and gender (particularly males over 85 years of age);
- recent upsetting events or problems;
- reports of low mood/feelings that life is not worth living;
- difficulty seeing solutions to problems;
- thoughts of death (suicidal ideation);
- competing stressors;
- recent or past suicide attempts;
- Lack of a support network (or withdrawing from them);
- a belief that there is no other way to resolve problems;
- an overwhelming sense of hopelessness or despair;
- decline in cognition and problem solving abilities;
- the presence of a plan and access to the means to carry out the plan.

Mental health problems, particularly depression, and other factors such as loss, illness, disability and lack of social support, sensory impair-ment and being a long time carer are all noted to contribute to suicide risk in older people (Butcher and McGonigal-Kennedy, 2005, p.54).

Interventions for suicidal ideation/attempts

The level of intervention required is based on the assessment of risk and what protective factors are available. Intervention options may include:

- monitoring and observing the person closely (if hospitalised);
- facilitating the development of, and providing coping strategies and opportunities to ventilate, distress;
- offering reassurance and emotional and other support;
- reviewing and coordinating current services and addressing carers' needs;
- facilitating increased community participation and reducing social isolation;
- increasing visits or phone contact by service providers or community support programs; and
- facilitating greater General Practitioner (GP) involvement.

Responsiveness to early indicators of depression is seen as one of the most effective suicide prevention strategies for older people.

Psychosis

Psychotic disorders of late life include first presentation psychosis in old age and early onset and late onset schizophrenia. 'Psychosis' can be defined as a loss of reality testing along with impaired mental functioning (Sadock, et al., 2007, p.272) and may include:

- Presence of delusions and/or hallucinations in the absence of insight;
- *Positive symptoms* or first ranked symptoms (as described by Kurt Schneider, cited in Fortinash, 2004, p.238) of schizophrenia, such as disorganised speech and grossly disorganised or catatonic behaviour;
- Negative symptoms or second ranked symptoms (as described by Kurt Schneider, cited in Fortinash, 2004, p.238), which may include restricted range and intensity of emotional expression (affective flattening), fluency and productivity of thought, empty, brief speech (alogia), decreased goal-driven behaviour (avolition) and loss of interest and enjoyment in activities (anhedonia). These symptoms should be distinguished from reactions to positive symptoms (fear and withdrawal), the sedating effects of medications, mood disorder and environmental under-stimulation.

Risk factors for late life schizophrenia

Risk factors include cognitive and sensory impairment, early life trauma, social isolation, being female and a family history of schizophrenia or affective disorder (Hassett et al., 2005).

Types of psychotic illness

Schizophrenia

Schizophrenia means 'split mindedness' and is referred to as a disorder of thought (Fortinash, 2007, p.237), with delusions and hallucinations common features of this psychotic illness.

Late-onset schizophrenia

Onset usually occurs after 45 years of age and runs a chronic course. There is a higher incidence in women, and sufferers tend to have better occupational history and tend to be married. Symptoms include paranoid delusions and hallucinations, but sufferers are less likely to have negative symptoms. Sensory deficits (hearing) are, however, common.

Schizoaffective Disorder

Schizoaffective Disorder generally occurs in late life and is characterised by affective symptoms which may include depressed mood (Fortinash, 2004, p.254), anhedonia, exaggerated or unrealistic ideas of guilt and worthlessness and somatic or nihilistic delusions.

Delusional disorders

In delusional disorders there are non-bizarre delusions, and hallucinations may not be prominent or may be related to the delusion. Functioning and behaviour may not otherwise be impaired. Erotomanic, grandiose, jealous, persecutory or somatic type delusions are often present. Patients may become litigious, withdrawn, angry or violent. Pre-morbidly clients are often obsessive, schizoid, paranoid or avoidant.

Charles-Bonet Syndrome

In Charles-Bonet Syndrome there is a spontaneous phenomenon of colourful, well-formed visual hallucinations without an auditory component. Often the patient has insight and may not be frightened of them, believing their eyesight is tricking them. It occurs more commonly in older people and initially it may be thought that the person is suffering from dementia, delirium or a substance abuse disorder (Jacob, Prasad, Boggild and Chandratre, 2004).

Interventions for older adults experiencing a psychosis

When interacting with the person (especially if they hold persecutory beliefs):

- Avoid arguing, scolding or negating the person's beliefs;

- Accept that the beliefs are real to the person but avoid accepting them, empathise with the experience and acknowledge their feelings (e.g. they may be feeling anxious about being in hospital);
- Respond to the underlying feelings behind the fears and beliefs;
- Gentle reality testing may be helpful if a trusting relationship has been established;
- Explain everything and be honest, open and respectful;
- Avoid being too friendly, overly familiar or inquisitive;
- Avoid using humour or light-hearted banter;
- More practically, offer choices in daily living and investigate suspicions to ensure that they are indeed unfounded;
- Check and correct hearing and vision if impaired; and
- Facilitate predictable routines and ensure consistency of carers (e.g. nurses who are providing care).

If the person experiences hallucinations, consider the response to hallucinatory phenomena. If the person enjoys their hallucinations, and if the phenomenon does not interfere with functioning and the person does not act in response to them, there may be little justification for intervening. Irrational outbursts, fear reactions or goal directed activity may be explained by visual or auditory phenomena. Any confounding trigger in the environment (e.g. loud television or radio) should be identified and minimised. Communication should be clear and unambiguous. Cautious reality testing and assisting the person to distinguish hallucinatory phenomena may relieve fear or distress.

The quiet and withdrawn person should be approached with an accepting attitude and the nurse should communicate a willingness to talk or listen when the person is ready. Reality orientation may be helpful to assist with day-to-day functioning. Hearing and vision should be maximised as much as possible. Appropriate meaningful activity and sensory stimulation may decrease the intensity of hallucinatory phenomena.

Inpatient admission may need to be considered if behavioural and psychosocial interventions have been unhelpful and/or treatment attempts unsuccessful. Admission should involve a comprehensive medical and neurological assessment, accurate identification of co-morbid psychopathology, evaluation of drug toxicity and a thorough history of previous management using psychotropic medication trials.

Mental health assessment of older people

When considering nursing assessment of an older person with mental health problems it is important to remember that assessment is a process, not an event, where information is obtained over time rather than in a brief visit or interaction. It is important also to be very clear what the presenting problem is and the reasons for conducting the assessment. Because of the impact of mental health problems on the older person's physical, psychological and social functioning, it is imperative that the assessment be biopsychosocial in nature (Hazelton, 2001, pp.96-97). Assessment will usually need to be multi-disciplinary because of effects of the ageing process, presence of physical illness, psychological reactions to illness/disability, atypical presentations, psychiatric manifestations of physical illness and the impact of environmental and social variables.

The development of a relationship between the mental health nurse and the older person is critical if assessment and interventions are to be in any way helpful or therapeutic. Important considerations are:

- believing the person will derive some benefit, whether a 'cure' or some improvement in functioning or perceived quality of life is fully achieved;
- taking sufficient time to develop the nurse-patient/client relationship;
- having an attitude that you believe the person is deserving of time, respect and courtesy, listening and understanding;
- avoiding technical language;
- avoiding communication and language that is dehumanising or patronising;
- using appropriate eye contact and names/titles, and
- avoiding too many direct or closed questions.

A comprehensive assessment by a specialist mental health service for older people would include the following:

- Medical history (especially psychiatric/neurological/medical);
- Previousillnesses(psychiatric/medical/neurological, substance use and abuse);
- Medication history (including over the counter drugs);

• History of present illnesses (including onset, course and precipitants);

- Social history (including pre-morbid personality traits, occupations, education, marital or significant relationships, children, living situation, religion, social activity and legal history);
- Mental State Examination (including cognitive screening such as MMSE or RUDAS);
- Health and functional needs assessment (including: nutritional status, sleep patterns, mobility/falls history, sensory deficits, pain behaviour, medication management, activities of daily living (ADLs) and any incontinence. It is important to note any changes from previous levels of functioning and timeframes associated with any identified changes);
- Pathology tests, recent X-rays or CT scans, blood screens and urine tests;
- Physical assessment and observations (including vital signs, temperature, pulse, blood pressure, respirations and weight);

- Caregiver resources (including problems undertaking the role, knowledge deficits, management strategies used, stress levels and coping mechanisms); and
- Information about the person's environment (including type, safety issues, functionality, possible isolation and satisfaction with and suitability of the environment in which they are residing or in which they are being cared for).

Common language and the use of standard measures such as cognitive screens, functional assessment tools and symptom-rating scales enhance cross-disciplinary communication.

Measuring outcomes used to assess older people's mental health

Assessment instruments (scales/tools) measure the responses to various items within a set of standardised questions (Tansella and Thornicroft, 2001, p.228). This results in a 'measurable outcome' where positive and negative changes in scores can be monitored by repeating the same measure at different intervals during the period of illness.

There are many outcome measurement scales for older people which enable the nurse and others to measure older adults' social functioning, quality of life, carer burden, consumer outcomes and depression, to name but a few. Outcome measures may be used by a clinician or self-reported by consumers. Slade refers to authors who suggest that 'outcomes should be considered multi-dimensionally, by measuring multiple outcome domains' (Slade, 2002, p.1339).

In mental illness there has been a shift towards measuring older adults' symptoms and social functioning and quality of life (Tansella and Thornicroft, 2001, p.172). Thus the goal when assessing people with mental illness may be to lessen symptom severity and improve functioning and their quality of life (Tansella and Thornicroft, 2001, p.172).

The appropriateness of the outcome measure to be used for older people should be considered in light of the client's cultural background, language, comprehension of difficulties being experienced and possible impaired senses and levels of disability (Newman, Kellett and Beail, 2003; Hibberd and Hong, 2007, p.248). An outcome measurement (of some type) should be conducted as part of the assessment process where information and a history of the phenomenology of the illness and the patient are recorded along with a general set of observations.

Assessment and outcome tools used in older persons' mental health

Achieving accurate outcome data in older person's mental health, particularly where self-reported measures are provided, can often be difficult due to consumer compliance, sensory impairment, communication difficulties and cognitive status. Nevertheless, it is important that when data is collected about patients we use it in some practical way to assist in improving the older adult's health outcomes (Ackland and Catford, 2004, pp.70-71) and assisting their family or carer.

The collection of a set of standardised outcome measures for mental health services across the lifespan has been required in Australia since 2001. Prominent among these measures are the Health of a Nation Outcome Scale (HoNOS), developed to measure health outcomes in the mentally ill (Pirkis, Burgess, Kirk, Dodson, Coombes and Williamson, 2005; Audin, Margison, Clark and Barkham, 2001), and the HoNOS 65+, specifically designed for clinical use with the elderly (Burns, et al., 1999). HoNOS is reported to have good validity, reliability, sensitivity to change and feasibility/utility (Pirkis et al., 2005). The clinical utility of measuring and recording outcome measures (particularly HoNOS 65+) in older people with mental health problems has been demonstrated by McKay and McDonald (2008).

Health of a Nation Outcome Scale 65+

HoNOS 65+, for use in older people, is a 12-item scale designed to gather additional information about physical problems and cognitive impairment across the four domains of impairment, behaviour, symptomatology and social functioning in the older person

(Burns et al., 1999). HoNOS 65+ is a clinician rated scale, with scores ranging from 0 to 4; a score of 2 or more being clinically significant and requiring further review and or treatment. The rating period of all HoNOS scoring is the previous two weeks.

HoNOS 65+ is a tool, easily completed as part of routine clinical practice (Burns et al., 1999), that can be used to consider the underlying determinants of the person's health status and assist in formulating evidence-based best practice. Within the 12 'key items', and from the domains noted previously, HoNOS 65+ offers knowledge about the client's:

- Degree of behaviour;
- Psychological state, including cognition;
- Physical state;
- Functional capacity (e.g. activities of daily living (ADLs) and occupational capacity);
- Living conditions; and
- Problems with relationships.

This encompasses all the elements of a biopsychosocial assessment. By considering each of the HoNOS 65+ individual scores clinicians can 'construct' the knowledge base needed to inform them of not only the client's degree of disability, but possibly (and more importantly for older patients) also those skills or items not affected during the period of illness. This allows nurses (and other clinicians) to focus on areas of concern in order to assist in the most appropriate intervention, designed to assist the recovery of that client and to enhance the remaining skills (Newman,

Kellett and Beail, 2003) and to monitor patient change for that episode of care (Slade, 2002, p.1341). This process reflects the opportunity to implement effective clinical management and for clinicians to use HoNOS 65+ (and other outcome measures) ‘ as an outcome indicator to guide the treatment of specific patients’ (Andrew and Page, 2005).

Other screening tools used in aged care

Standardised screening tools can be used in non-specialist settings to screen for cognitive impairment, depression and delirium. The Mental State Examination (MSE) is an essential component of the mental health assessment of an older person. The MSE, undertaken at assessment, provides a baseline description of a person’s present appearance, demeanour, speech, actions and thoughts (Hazelton, 2001, p.97). Other more specific assessment tools used in older person mental health include:

Mini-Mental State Examination (MMSE)

The Mini-Mental State Examination (MMSE) (Folstein et al., 1975) is a quick and widely known screening tool for measuring whether any degree of cognitive impairment is present. The tool has 30 questions measuring orientation, attention and calculation capabilities, language, recall and perception. While not a comprehensive assessment, it is used in a variety of settings by specialists, non-specialists and students. A score of less than 24 indicates a degree of cognitive impairment, suggesting that further investigation is required (Murphy, 2004, p.336.).

Used independently of the MMSE, the clock-drawing test (Shulman, 2000) is a simple, non-threatening cognitive screen which can provide a wealth of information about executive functions, such as planning, as well as constructional apraxia (the inability to put together objects in their correct spatial relationship to each other) and is useful when the patient may be unable, for various reasons (e.g. suspiciousness), to cope with a full MMSE.

Rowland Universal Dementia Assessment Scale

The Rowland Universal Dementia Assessment Scale (RUDAS) has been developed in Australia for use among ethnically diverse communities (Rowland et al., 2000). It is used as an alternative to the MMSE and results are less influenced by language, education and gender.

Geriatric Depression Scale (GDS)

The Geriatric Depression Scale is commonly used in clinical practice with two versions available: the

15- and 30-item scales (Yesavage, 1993). The 15-item GDS is a shortened version used to detect depressive symptoms and can be used to monitor changes in depression during treatment. Participants respond to questions by answering 'Yes' or 'No' about how they feel. The GDS should not be used with cognitively impaired older adults. A score greater than five in the 15 item scale indicates possible depression and requires further assessment and diagnostic evaluation (Murphy, 2004, p.336).

Cornell Scale for Depression in Dementia

The Cornell Scale for Depression in Dementia is a 19-item scale for identification of depressive symptoms in dementia. Items are scored by observing as well as gaining information from others. It is a 3-point scale scored as: Absent (0), Mild (1), Severe (2), for a total of a possible 38 points (Sharp et al., 2002). Scores above 18 indicate definite depression. Scores below 6 indicate absence of significant depressive symptoms (Australian Government, 2005).

Confusion Assessment Method

The Confusion Assessment Method (CAM) is a screening tool for delirium which identifies four key components: (1) acute onset or fluctuation of symptoms, (2) inattention, (3) disorganised thinking and (4) consciousness (Inouye et al., 1990).

Clinical utility of outcome measures and screening tools

Knowledge generated from outcome measures can be useful for the client and for clinicians. They offer an opportunity to set goals according to the identified areas of deficit in collaboration with the client (where possible), carer and clinician. For the client this knowledge offers a template for planning interventions, assists in monitoring progress, provides feedback, guides actions for rehabilitation and enhanced recovery and offers opportunities to confirm the effectiveness of the goals set and the compliance with interventions undertaken. For the nurse and other health professionals this knowledge focuses on the 'holistic' needs of the client as opposed to only the medical or psychiatric issues. It provides a structured means of information gathering that helps ensure a systematic approach to patient care, encouraging nurses to consider the phenomenology of that person allowing for a greater understanding of the client and their life experiences past and present. It also offers nurses (and others) the opportunity to measure the outcomes and effectiveness of the agreed plan of care (Burns et al., 1999).

Mental health promotion

Mental health promotion is about maximising the older adult's mental health and improving feelings of wellbeing (Commonwealth Department of Health and Aged Care, 2000, p.6). Promoting good mental health for older people includes providing emotional and physical support, preventing decline and enhancing the older person's remaining attributes.

The phenomenon of the ageing population has generated social and public health debate. It is important, therefore, to identify priorities for health promotion programs and health promotion research for older adults, as highlighted by Howart, Duncan and Horner (2004). Promoting physical and mental health are key components of better health and longer life expectancy (Mendes de Leon, Glass and Berkman, 2003; Uchino, 2006). Howart et al. (2004, p.50) suggest that increasing the health status of older people should be given increased importance. Risk factors for developing a mental illness among the elderly are many and include physical impairment, chronic ill health, cognitive decline, unresolved loss and grief, social isolation and a lack of social networks and support systems. However, protective factors are also many and include good health, reliable and consistent support networks and connectiveness and companionship with friends and family (McDonald and Brown, 2008; Turvey, et al., 2002; Commonwealth Department of Health and Aged Care, 2000).

Social supports are important when assessing factors that will promote wellbeing, particularly among older adults (Hansson, 2006). A study by McDonald and Brown (2008) describes the significant benefits of social support and social networking through group participation by older adults, with and without mental health problems, and highlighted group membership and peer support as a positive means for supporting recovery and promoting positive emotional health and wellbeing for older people.

Referral

Referral to an appropriate mental health service and mobilising other supports is required for the person for whom suicide ideation is present and persistent or associated with features of depressive or other mental health problems.

Referral to hospital-based care is required for those:

- who are at high or immediate risk;
- who have little support within the community or access to services;
- who are at risk of harm to self or others, experiencing severe despair or depression;
- who are at need of a clear diagnosis; or
- for whom in-patient treatment is required for medical problems.

Some older adults requiring admission may necessitate scheduling under the Mental Health Act (involuntary admission) or the Guardianship Act.

Conclusion

Mental illness is a significant problem in the elderly. Specialist mental health services for older people and specialist clinicians, including nurses, have evolved over many years to better manage the needs of this often complex group of consumers. However, important to the end result of older people's illness experience is the need for them to have a say in how care progams, treatment options and services are delivered in order to achieve the most favourable outcome. Interestingly, Ames and Ritchie (2007, p.453) propose that a changing profile of educated and more assertive older adults should be anticipated in the future. This cohort will have knowledge of and expect access to health and social services as required and their expectation of and satisfaction with appropriate service delivery will be different.

Reflective questions:

1) Describe the social determinants of health for older people.
2) Explore the risk factors for developing a mental health problem in old age.
3) Evaluate psychosocial interventions for the management of mental health problems in the elderly.
4) Evaluate the screening tool used in assessment of the older person.

5) What are the benefits of measuring outcomes in mental health of older people?
6) Discuss the part that health promotion plays in the mental health of older people.

Chapter 10

Clinical pharmacology and older adults

Dr. Pascale Dettwiller, DPharm., MHumanBiol., Cert. Grtre, Pharm., AACPA
Associate Professor of Pharmacy, Discipline Leader, SELS, CDU

Objectives:

This chapter will enable the reader to:

1) Demonstrate why clinical pharmacology has significant implications for older adults;
2) Conduct an assessment of the medications that an older adult is currently taking;
3) Identify why an assessment of over-the-counter medications is also important;
4) Define pharmacokinetics and pharmacodynamics;
5) Describe the impact of ageing on drug absorption, distribution, metabolism and elimination; and
6) Define polypharmacy, non-compliance, adverse drug reactions, extrapyramidal side effects and neuroleptic malignant syndrome.

Introduction

In an increasing ageing population, inappropriate medication management of older adults with chronic clinical conditions can lead to real risks for their safety and for the safety of health care staff. The elderly population is consuming a significant number of medications, a major part of these being given on prescription by medical practitioners. Many older adults are being given more than one drug at any one time and polypharmacy is used to characterise the situation where more than five drugs are prescribed at any one time (Hilmer, 2008). There are, however, prescription and/or non-prescription drugs (over-the-counter drugs, diet supplements, complementary and alternative medicines) taken by older people without the knowledge of their current General Practitioner (GP). Another major issue arises when older adults are admitted to hospital and then discharged; many medication regimes are changed during hospitalisation or altered on discharge, and the older adult patient does not know for what purpose the new drugs are being taken. Polypharmaceutical prescribing may then affect compliance. It is important to note that polypharmacy also contributes to an increase of adverse drug events, including drug-disease interactions and drug-drug interactions (Pirmohamed, James, Meakin, Green, Scott, Walley, Farrar, Park and Breckenridge, 2004).

Are older adults to be considered as 'special' when it comes to medication? Chronological age on its own may not be an appropriate way to categorise older adults (this concept was discussed in Chapter 2 by Dr. Mary MacGibbon). In general, those adults over 65 years (and over 50 years for Aboriginal and Torres Strait Islander people) are often described as aged, older or elderly. However, there is no widely accepted name for, or definition of, an older adult (AMH, Aged care, 2006). While a person's age should not affect treatment objectives, they can be affected by several phenomena that are more prevalent with increasing age, for example, modification in pharmacokinetics and pharmacodynamics occur with normal ageing chronology. These changes will be discussed later in this chapter. It is important to mention that if the types of adverse events (e.g. adverse drug reactions) are similar to those of other adults, the intensity and frequency is often more severe. This is a contributing factor to increased hospitalisation and multiple medication changes (Halter, 2009).

Medication questionnaire for older adults

Assessment of the older adult will include careful consideration of the medications they are taking. A medication questionnaire may assist in this assessment. By looking through various textbooks, it is clear that several examples of medication questionnaires can be found. The following are some questions that should perhaps be considered:

1) What medications do you take?
2) Do you know why you take each medication?
3) Do you know when you started taking each medication?
4) How often do you take each medication and how many of each medication do you take?
5) Have you ever experienced any adverse effects to any of your medications?
6) Have you noticed any changes in your health since beginning taking any of your medications?
7) Do you follow any special health care practices? Do you have a management plan?
8) How many doctors have you seen in the past 12 months?
9) Do you experience any difficulties in obtaining your medications?
10) Do you have any difficulties in complying with your medications and if so what kind?
11) Do you have any difficulties in swallowing some of your medications?
12) What health care problems are you presently experiencing for which you have been prescribed medications?

For a more comprehensive checklist for older adults' medication history see Checklist for Pharmaceutical Society of Australia (http://www.psa.org.au/site.php?id=3445).

In addition to the medications prescribed by the patient's doctor, one should also ask about any over-the-counter (OTC) medications, diet supplements, 'complementary' and/or alternative medicines. Commonly, older individuals (two thirds of older adults over 65 years) may take OTC medications for gastrointestinal tract (GIT) problems (e.g. constipation), pain relief (e.g. arthritis or back pain) or self-administered medications (e.g. cough and cold medicines, eye drops, etc.). The most commonly used OTC medications include analgesics, antacids, cough and cold medicines and laxatives (Merck Manual a.).

Some analgesics (e.g. non-steroidal analgesics (NSAIDs)) can alter blood coagulation properties and can cause gastric irritation and therefore GIT bleeding. Due to contributing factors in altering kidney function, this class of analgesics (NSAIDs) is implicated in the development of confusion, irritability, diarrhoea, hypothermia and hearing and vision disturbances in older adults. Paracetamol is the first choice for pain relief because it is safer than NSAIDs while still being effective. Nevertheless, paracetamol should be used cautiously in older adults with liver disease (not to exceed 4g/day) and in those who consume more than two alcoholic drinks per day because of the increased risk of hepatotoxicity (National Prescribing Service Ltd., 2007; Halter, 2009).

Laxatives may result in a 'lazy' bowel, interfere with absorption of nutrients (liposoluble ADEK vitamins) and fluids re-absorption (water and electrolytes), and may also cause weight loss and weakness in the elderly (Pharmacy Guild of Australia, http ://www.novapolic y.com/pccp/PDF/MODULES-MEDICATION_AND_CONTINENCE.pdf; Halter, 2009). Antacids decrease absorption of psychoactive drugs and nutrients, by delaying gastric emptying, and absorption of digoxin. Antacids also increase antibiotic absorption and may cause constipation or diarrhoea. Vitamin supplements may be helpful for older adults generally but may contribute to constipation when they contain iron, while vitamin C may cause kidney stones. Some cough preparations may alter blood pressure and precipitate psychiatric symptoms; antihistamine based medications have been shown to cause paradoxical reactions such as agitation and excitement (Ratnaike, 2000; Halter, 2009).

Pharmacokinetics

Age-related changes and disease-related alterations affecting organ functioning can affect drug pharmacokinetics in older adults (Barry and Cusack, 2004). Pharmacokinetic processes determine the relationship between drug input (dosage, dosage form, frequency, route of administration, etc.) and the concentration of drug achieved over time. Pharmacokinetics describes the time course by which the body Absorbs a medication and Distributes it, how it is activated through Metabolism, and how it is Excreted (ADME) (Noble, 2003). An increase of inter-individual variability is the main change in pharmacokinetics associated with ageing (Burton, 2006).

Absorption

Absorption describes how and where the drug enters the body and moves into the systemic blood circulation and lymphatic systems. Drug absorption can commonly be altered in older adults due to various physiological changes including gastric pH increase, making it more alkaline, gastric emptying slows, increase in duodenal diverticuli and decrease in small-bowel surface (Merck Manual b.). The presence or absence of nutrients may also affect absorption and gastric emptying. Changes might be quite significant for some drugs which require a more acidic pH for absorption (e.g. aspirin, penicillin). Changes in drug absorption, however, do tend to be trivial and therefore in the main clinically inconsequential (Halter, 2009).

Distribution

Changes in volume of distribution affect the half-life of drugs and the loading dose in the following ways:

a) With ageing, there is a decrease in total body fluid and body mass and a significant increase in total body fat. Distribution of drugs will vary depending on their physicochemical properties (Merck Manual c.). Lipophilic drugs such as benzodiazepines (e.g. temazepam, nitrazepam, diazepam, etc.) and anti-psychotics (haloperidol) will be released from adipose tissue more slowly, causing a prolonged release effect that may lead to residual drowsiness and increased risk of falls. Water-soluble drugs (e.g. digoxin) may display an increased blood and tissue concentration (Mangoni and Jackson, 2004; Patient UK, 2008);

b) Ageing affects plasma proteins concentration (serum albumin and alpha-1 acid glycoprotein) significantly. Serum albumin hepatic production is reduced by 19% in older adults and drugs highly binding to serum albumin (e.g. digoxin, phenytoin, warfarin, hormones, AGIIRB, clopidogrel, sertraline, diazepam, diclofenac, etc.) will compete with each other for transport receptor sites, thereby freeing more drugs to interact with other medications (Ebersole, Hess, Toughy and Jet, 2008). Albumin is commonly reduced in malnutrition and acute illness (Mangoni and Jackson, 2004). This contributes to the increase of adverse events recorded in older adults; and

c) In older adults with acute disease or malnutrition, there can be rapid decreases in the serum albumin level, which may enhance drug effects. This is because serum concentrations of unbound drugs are increased until metabolic excretion compensation occurs.

Metabolism

There is reduced hepatic mass and hepatic blood flow with ageing, which affects the hepatic elimination of drugs (Wynne, 2005). The liver is the main organ responsible for medication metabolism. The first pass metabolism leads to an increased bioavailability of drug that undergoes significant first pass metabolism and decreased activation of 'prodrugs'; the drugs affected include: pethidine, amitryptiline, diazepam, morphine, codeine, verapamil, diclofenac, paracetamol, atorvastatin, etc. (Hilmer, Shenfield and Le Couteur, 2005).

Accumulation of metabolites increases the risk of toxicity in older adults due to age-related decreases in renal clearance, unless the maintenance doses are reduced (Davison, Cameron, Grunfeld, Ponticelli, Ritz, Winearls and van Persele, 2005).

Elimination

Renal mass and renal blood flow decrease significantly with age such that glomerular filtration rate should be evaluated before commencing a medication regime (Merle, Laroche, Dantoine and Charmes, 2005). The reduction in glomerular filtration rate (GFR) results in an accumulation of medications and their toxic meta-bolites. Interestingly, serum creatinine levels may remain within normal limits because older adults have less lean body mass and produce less creatinine. This is especially important with narrow therapeutic index drugs such as digoxin, lithium and gentamicin (Mangoni and Jackson, 2004). This is likely to result in serious adverse effects.

Drugs that are likely to be affected by renal changes include digoxin, ranitidine, amantadine and lithium. The dose of these drugs given long term should be reviewed periodically.

Acute illness (myocardial infarction, urinary tract infections, etc.) can lead to a rapid decrease in renal function, requiring prompt drug adjustment. Reduction in drug elimination is more pronounced in malnourished and frail older adults (Turnheim, 2003).

Altered pharmacodynamics in the elderly

Pharmacodynamics refers to the time course and the effect of medications on cellular and organ function. It is important to note that it is difficult to predict response variation due to the wide interindividual heterogeneity (Halter, 2009; Burton, 2006). In older adults, the effects of similar drug concentration at the site of action may display:

1) Increased sensitivity to some drugs due to changes in number of receptors and/or affinity,

receptors alteration or decreased homeostatic mechanisms (feedback regulations which contribute to secondary compensatory mechanisms). This may predispose some to adverse drug events (Bressler and Bahl, 2003). Hypnotics, anti-depressants, benzodiazepines, heparin, levodopa, morphine and warfarin can all be included in this category;

2) Decreased sensitivity to beta blockers (dopamine) (Woodward, Elliott, Vernon, Tanner and Saunders, 2006); and
3) Decreased and/or increased sensitivity to calcium channel blockers (e.g. nifedipine) (Boon, Colledge and Walker, 2006).

Drugs commonly cause changes in behaviour among the elderly (AMH, Aged Care 2006). Changes include:

1) Incontinence (benzodiazepines, diuretics);
2) Confusion (antibiotics, digoxin, NSAIDs);
3) Falls (anti-psychotics, anti-hypertensive drugs);
4) Depression (anti-arthritics, anxiolytics);
5) Sexual dysfunction (anti-psychotics, anti-depressants); and
6) Mobility problems (anxiolytics, anti-psychotics).

Other factors that affect medications in older adults

As we have already seen, pharmacokinetic and pharmacodynamic effects influence the effectiveness of medications in older individuals, but weight and gender also have an impact. Body size, for example, affects volume of distribution, therapeutic and adverse drug reactions associated with medications. Older people who are small or who have lost weight may be more susceptible to adverse drug events. Older women are at a higher risk for altered therapeutic effects and adverse drug events. Women use more prescribed drugs than men and women will also self-medicate more readily (Miller, 2004).

You should identify physiological factors in women such as smaller size (compared to men), hormonal influences, higher proportion of body fat to lean body tissue and socioeconomic factors.

Additional comments:

Pathological processes in the presence of functional impairments may also influence the effects of medication in older adults. For example, disease processes may exacerbate agerelated change. Sub-nutritional states in the elderly may decrease serum albumin levels while congestive cardiac failure may decrease the metabolism and excretion of medications. Adverse drug events may affect disease processes. Anticholinerics may exacerbate prostatic hypertrophy and lead to urinary retention (Miller, 2004).

Myths about medications perpetuated among older people may also affect the therapeutic effect of medication. For example, OTC medications may be seen as providing a 'quick fix' and save the older person going to the doctor. Prescriptions, on the other hand, may be seen as providing a 'cure' for conditions that may be incurable. Alternatively, prescriptions may be seen as being more effective when a non-medication remedy would be preferable. Other older people may think that they can stop taking their antibiotics once they have, for example, stopped coughing.

Communication barriers may include not questioning the prescriber about the prescribed medication or about the need to take the medication, as the older person often perceives their GP as knowing best. Sometimes prescribers may not discuss the older person's medication regimen due to a lack of ability to understand; this is particularly so where the regimen is a complex one. Hearing, language barriers and other impairments may also affect the medical plan. Physiological or pathological changes in swallowing ability for older adults need to be assessed as this has the potential to lead to dose delivery problems (Beardsley, Kimberlin and Tindall, 2007).

Medication effects in older individuals may not be well understood by the medical practitioners and there is a need to be cautious when prescribing multiple medications for older people.

Inappropriate medication prescribing practices for older adults has also been noted in the literature. The problem occurs particularly in residential care settings (see below). These problems relate to the under-use and over-use of medications.

Polypharmacy refers to the use of multiple medications (more than five), and these may come from multiple sources (Junius-Walker, Theile and Hummers-Pradier, 2007). The presence of multiple illnesses in older adults may not be the only reason. Polypharmacy increases the risk of noncompliance and adverse drug events. A complex medication regimen for multiple illnesses requires diligent clinical and biological monitoring.

Non-compliance describes any person who is not following medication management plans, missing doses, not filling prescriptions, taking medications irregularly and/or at inappropriate times, forgetting to take them or mixing them with inappropriate food or drinks (George, Kong, Thoman and Stewart, 2005).

Hearing and vision impairment, memory loss, dexterity problems, lack of supervision, economic situation, lack of transport, problems of social isolation, literacy levels and lack of knowledge or understanding of complex issues such as drug regimes and their side effects are all compelling reasons/indicators for non-compliance.

What are some possible solutions to the problems of non-compliance?*

[*Anti-psychotic medication should not be given to residents with Lewy Body Dementia or Parkinson's disease (Royal Australian College of General Practitioners, 2005).]

Insufficient recognition of adverse drug events

Adverse drug events in older adults may be misinterpreted or go unrecognised. One reason for this may be the misinterpretation of signs as age-related changes or the development of underlying pathological conditions. Moreover, drug side effects may be mistaken for the onset of a new illness. Although not uncommon in other age groups, adverse drug events occur more commonly in older adults (Roughead, 2005).

Drugs and Nursing Home Residents

Between 20% and 50% of residents in aged care facilities are prescribed one or more psychotropic medication. Psychotropic medications should only be prescribed to target specific symptoms (Hunter Division of General Practice, 2007).

In a study by Snowdon (2006), psychotropic drugs were shown to be more likely to be given to those nursing home residents with greater cognitive impairment and with more disturbed behaviour. Psychotropics include anti-psychotics, anxiolytics, sedative-hypnotics, anti-depressants, and anti-manic drugs (mood stabilisers). Remarkably, at least half of antidepressant doses were sub-therapeutic.

The use of psychotropic medication in residential aged care facilities should only be used where:

1) There is no physical cause for the behaviour;
2) It is unrelated to administration of other medication (e.g. adverse effect caused by another drug); and
3) The older resident is not a candidate for, or has not responded to, non-pharmacological intervention (behaviour modification approach, music therapy, etc.).

Psychotropic medication may be used in geriatrics for depression, schizophrenia, bipolar affective disorder, dementia and Parkinson's disease. It should be noted that typical anti-psychotic medications (e.g. chlorpromazine, trifluoperazine, haloperidol) may also cause extra-pyramidal side effects (EPSEs), although atypical anti-psychotics (e.g. clozapine, risperidone, olanzapine) may have lower propensity for causing EPSEs (Australian Government, 2007). EPSEs include tremor, akathisia, slurred speech, dystonia, bradykinesia and rigidity (Read and Purse, 2009).

Neuroleptic Malignant Syndrome (NMS) represents a serious and potentially lethal drug reaction to anti-psychotics. It is however, uncommon. NMS is found in both genders and all ages. All classes of drugs that induce dopamine-2 receptor blockade have been associated with the syndrome, and this includes both typical and atypical anti-psychotic agents (e.g. olanzapine; clozapine) (Australian Government, 2007).

NMS presents a rare but serious risk of mortality. Primary symptoms include:

- Muscle rigidity;
- Hyperreflexia;
- Sudden high fever (hyperthermia);
- Sweating and shivering;
- Agitation;
- Dysrhythmias (Tachycardia);
- Fluctuations in blood pressure;
- Rise and fall in level of consciousness;
- Changes in mental state (e.g. confusion);
- Seizures or coma; and
- Death from cardio-vascular collapse. (Carmela and Ernest, 2007; Isbister, Buckley and Whyte, 2007)

Treatment includes withdrawal of anti-psychotic medication, anti-pyretics, fluids and muscle relaxants (Isbister, Buckley and Whyte, 2007).

A regular pharmacist review of medications prescribed for older adults in residential care facilities has the potential to reduce the number of medicines prescribed and to have a positive impact on morbidity and mortality (Australian Government, 2008).

Clinical guidelines

It is important to take a patient's medication history (including dose, formulation, etc.) and to note their reactions to previously administered drugs. Consider what are the most accurate diagnoses and concurrent illnesses. Symptoms should be targeted and responses monitored accordingly. Generally, medications for older adults are ordered at one third to one half of the dose recommended for adults or younger patients. Incremental dosing of older adults is a warranty to minimise adverse drug effects and to optimise individual treatments (e.g. patients should be on a dose of an anti-psychotic medication for at least three days prior to a dose increase, while the same should apply when reducing a dosing regimen) (Halter, 2009).

Prior to treating behaviours with medication, it is important to consider the following issues:

1) Does the symptom warrant drug treatment, and why?
2) Is the symptom/behaviour drug-responsive?
3) Which category of medication is most suitable for this symptom?
4) What are the predictable and potential side effects?
5) For how long should the treatment be continued?

Medication advice for older adult patients

- Encourage older adults to ask questions about their medications and provide them with written information such as the Consumer Medication Information (CMI).
- Encourage patients to write their questions down.
- When going to medical practitioners for assessment, advise patients to take a list of all their

medications with them and recommend a regular review of the medications.

- Encourage patients to tell their doctor if they have allergies or any adverse events to any listed medications.
- Recommend that a pharmacist perform at least one yearly home medication review of their medication regimen, as per Medicare and Department of Veterans Affairs entitlements.

References

Chapter 1

Abbey, J., Abbey, B., Bridges, P., Elder, R., Lemcke, P., Liddle, J. and Thornton, R. (2006). Clinical placements in residential aged care facilities: The impact on nursing students' perception of aged care and the effect on career plans. Australian Journal of Advanced Nursing, 23, 4, 14-19.

Allied and Scientific Health Office (2009). Health service framework for older people 2009-2016. South Australian Government. http://www.health.sa.gov.au /clinical_networks.

Australian Bureau of Statistics (2003). Population by age and sex.

Australian Bureau of Statistics (2004). Older people, New South Wales. 4108.1.

Australian Bureau of Statistics (2006). Census Tables: Indigenous Status by Age, Cat. No.2068.

Australian Government (2006). Aspects of retirement for older women. Australian Government Office.

Australian Government (2009). Community aged care packages. Department of Health and Ageing.

Australian Government Department of Health and Ageing. Aged care in Australia. http://www.agedcare australia.gov.au.

Australian Institute of Health and Welfare (2007). Older Australians at a glance. 2nd ed. Commonwealth of Australia.

Australia's older people. Demographic issues and population ageing. http://www.aic.gov.au/publications/rpp/32/older.pdf.

Barnett, A., Smith, B., Lord, S.R., Williams, M. and Baumand, A. (2003). Community-based exercise improves balance and reduces falls in at-risk older people: a randomised controlled trial. Age and Aging, 32, 407-414.

Bates, A., Donaldson, A., Lloyd, B., Castell, S., Krolik, P. And Coleman, R. (2009). Staying alive, staying strong: pilot evaluation of a once-weekly strength training program for older adults. Health Promotion Journal of Australia, 20, 1, 42-47.

Benevolent Society (2007). Ocean Street Project Information Sheet No.1. Downloaded from http://www.bensoc.org.au.

Birren, J.E. and Schaie, K.W. (Eds.) (2001)/. Handbook of the psychology of aging. 5th ed. San Diego: Academic Press.

Booth, H. And Tickle, L. (2003). The future aged: new projections of Australia's elderly population. Australasian Journal on Ageing, 22,4,196-202.

Bruen, W. (2005). Policy update. Aged care in Australia: past, present and future. Australasian Journal on Ageing, 24, 3, 130-133.

Burbank, P.M., Padula, C.A. and Nigg, C.R. (2000). Changing health behaviors of older adults. Journal of Gerontological Nursing, 26,3, 26-33.

Cattan, M., White, M., Bond, J. and Learmouth, A. (2005). Preventing social isolation and loneliness among older people: a systematic review of health promotion interventions. Aging & Society, 25, 41-67.

Courtney, M.D., Tong, S. and Walsh, A.M. (2000). Acute care nurses' attitudes toward older patients: a literature review. International Journal of Nursing Practice, 6, 2, 62-69.

Crandall, R.C. (1991). Gerontology: a behavioral science approach. 2nd ed. New York: McGraw-Hill.

Crowe, M. (1996). Health promotion needs of Aboriginal people. Australian Journal on Ageing, 15.1.11-13.

Demographic profile; Australia at a glance. http://www.aihw.gov.au/publications/age/oag04/oag04-c01.pdf.

Department of Health and Ageing (2008). Achievements in aged care – First anniversary report card. Downloaded http://health.gov.au.

Ebersole, P., Hess, P. and Luggen, A.S. (2004). Toward health aging. Human needs and nursing response. St. Louis, MO: Mosby.

Encel, S. And Studencki, H. (2004). Older workers: can they succeed in the job market. Australasian Journal on Ageing, 23, 1, 33-37.

Eliopoulos, C. (2004). Gerontological nursing. Lippincott Williams and Wilkins.

Geriaction (2000). Competency Standards for the Advanced Gerontological Nurse. Sydney: John Thrift Publishing.

Grabinski, C.J. (2007). 101 careers in gerontology. New York: Springer Publishing Company.

Henderson, J., Xiao, L., Siegloff, Kelton, M., and Paterson, J. (2008). 'Older people have lived their lives': First year nursing students' attitudes towards older people. Contemporary Nurse, 30, 1, 32-45.

Herdman, E. (2002). Challenging the discourses of nursing ageism. International Journal of Nursing Studies, 39, 105-114.

Hirvensalo, M., Heikkinen, E., Lintunen, T. and Rantanen, T. (2003). The effect of advice by health care professionals on increasing physical activity of older people. Scandinavian Journal of Medicine & Science in Sports, 13, 4, 231-236.

Imamura, E. (2002). Amy's chat room: health promotion programmes for community dwelling elderly adults. International Journal of Nursing Practice, 8,1 61-64.

Irizarry, C., West, D. and Downing, A. (2001). Use of the internet by older rural South Australians, 20,3, 153-155.

Joanna Briggs Institute for Evidence-Based Nursing and Midwifery (2001).

Koori Connections: Indigenous Equity Strategies, in Health Promotions Strategies, volume 6, Number 1, February, 2006. Department of Human Services, Victorian Government.

Lazonby, A. (2007). The changing face of the aged care sector in NZ, Working Paper. Retirement Policy and Research Centre.

Economics Department, University of Auckland.

Meiner, S.E. and Lueckenotte, A.G. (2006). Gerontologic nursing. 3rd ed. Missouri: Elsevier.

Miller, C.A. (2009). Nursing for wellness in older adults. 4th ed. Philadelphia: Lippincott Williams & Wilkins.

Ministry of Health (2002). Health of older people in New Zealand. A statistical reference. Wellington, New Zealand.

Murray, T.A. and Lewis, C. Community-based nursing care. In Brown, D. and Edwards, H., lewis, S.L., Heitkemper, M. McL., Dirksen, S.R., O'Brien, P.G. and Bucher, L. (2008). Lewis's medical-surgical nursing. Assessment and management of clinical problems. 2nd ed. Sydney: Mosby.

Parliament of Australia. 'Caring for the elderly' – an overview of aged care support and services in Australia. Parliamentary Library.

Parliament of Australia. Fertility: A baby bounce for Australia. Parliamentary Library.

Peel, N., Barlett, H. And McClure, R. (2004). Healthy ageing: how is it defined and measured? Australasian Journal on Ageing, 23, 3, 115-119.

Phillipson, C. History and historical sociology: Divergent paths in the study of ageing. Ageing and Society, 21, 507-522).

Phillipson, C. and Scharf, T. (2004). Research into ageing at Keele: Developing inter-disciplinary perspectives. www.keele.ac.uk/research/lcs/csg.

Population ageing in NZ (2006). http://www.google.com.au/search?hl=en&q=Population+ageing+in+N

Z-Stats+NZ+stat.govt.nz%2Fproducts-and-services%2FArticles%2Fpop-ageing-Feb00.htm.&btnG=Search&meta=.

Reed, J., Inglis, P., Cook, G., Clarke, C. and Cook, M. (2001). Specialist nurses for older people: implications from UK development sites. Journal of Advanced Nursing, 58, 4, 368-376.

Resnick, B. (2003). Health promotion practices of older adults: testing an individualized approach. Journal of Clinical Nursing, 12, 1, 46-55.

Richmond, D. & McCracken, H. (1996). Health promotion and education for the elderly: experience in an academic department of geriatric medicine. Australian Journal on Ageing, 15,1,18-21.

Richmond, R.L. (2008). The changing face of the Australian population: growth in centenarians. eMJA, 188, 12, 720-723.

Rognstad, M-K, Aasland, O. and Granum, V. (2004). How do nursing student regard their future career? Career preferences in the post-modern society. Nurse Education Today, 24, 493-500.

Russell, C., Campbell, A. And Hughes, I. (2008). Ageing, social capital and the internet: findings from an exploratory study of Australian 'silver surfers'. Australasian Journal on Ageing, 27,2,78-82.

Santrock, J.W. (2006). *Life-span development.* 10th ed. Boston: McGraw Hill.

Soderhamn, O., Lindencrona, C. and Gustavsson, S.M. (2001). Attitudes toward older people among nursing students and registered nurses in Sweden. Nurse Education Today, 21, 225-229.

Stanley, M. and Beare, P.G. (2005). Gerontological nursing. Philadelphia: F.A. Davis Company.

Statistics New Zealand. Older New Zealanders – 65 and beyond (2004). Wellington, New Zealand.

Statistics NZ. Demographic trends (a), 2007. Death and life expectancy. http://www.stats.govt.nz/analyticalreports/dem.trends-07/default.htm. Downloaded 18 July 2009.

Statistical NZ, Demographic trends (b), 2007. Census snapshot: Cultural diversity.stats.govt.nz/NR/872D2D96-78A346E1-A419-E2CDF3835D2/O/CenCulDiv.pdf.

Statistical NZ, Demographic trends (c), 2007. Population change and structure. http://www.stats.govt.nz/analyticalreports/dem.trends-07/default.htm. Downloaded 18 July 2009.

Stevens, J.A. & Crouch, M.W. (1992). Working with the elderly: do students care for it? The Australian Journal of Advanced Nursing, 9, 3, 12-17.

The Australian Centre on Ageing. Submission to the House of Representatives Employment and Workplace Relations Committee. Downloaded from http://www.aph.gov/au/HOUSE/committee/ewrwp/paidwork/subs/sub91.pdf.

The Medical News (2005). Why do women live longer than men? Liverpool John Moores University.

Wallace, C., Brown, P., Cumming, M. & Waugh, K. (2007). Teaching Nursing Home: Development of an Australian Model. Geriaction, 25, 3, 5-11.

Wright, T. Never say die. http://bulletin.ninemsn.com.au/bulletin/EdDesk.nsf/0/a5e622b02c5a0753ca256e4e000

Chapter 2

Aged Care Act & User Rights Principles (1997) accessed 4 November 2009at http://www.healthyactive.gov.au/internet/main/publishing.nsf.htm

Australian Nursing Federation (1997) *Competency Standards for the Advanced Nurse.* ANF, Canberra Commonwealth Department of Housing and Aged Care (1987) *Gazette S303 under National Health Act 1953.* AGPS, Canberra.

Department of Health and Ageing Working Group on Aged Care Worker Qualifications (2001) *Review of current role of ENs in aged care: Future directions Aged Care.* National Aged Care Forum, DOHA, Canberra.

Dept Community Services (1986) *Nursing Homes and Hostels Review.* AGPS, Canberra.

Dept Health and Ageing (2001) *Inquiry into Ageing over next 40 years.* DOHA, Canberra.

Dept Health and Ageing (2003) *Enrolled Nurse Working Party report,* ACENWP, DOHA, Canberra

Edwards, H. (2004) *Aged Care core Component in Undergraduate Nursing Curricula Principles Paper* Queensland University of Technology.

Federal Budget 2002-03, Paper 5. *Intergenerational Report.* Internet.

Gardiner, H. (2002) *Health Policy: Development, Implementation and Evaluation in Australia.* Churchill Livingstone, Melbourne.

Gray, G. (1993) *ANCI National Competencies for RNs and ENs in Recommended domains.* ANC, Canberra.

Gray, L. (2001) *Two Year Review of Aged Care Reforms.* DOHA, Canberra.

Hogwood, B.W. & Gunn, L.A. (1989) *Policy analysis for the real world.* Oxford University Press, Oxford. p.13-19.

Kalish, B.J. & Kalish, P.A. (1982) *Politics of Nursing* J.B. Lippincott, Philadelphia.

McDonald, T. (2005) *At What Cost? Aged care industry costs arising from Resident Classification Scheme processes.* October. Published on http://www.agedcareassociation.com.au (accessed 23 October 2009.

National Review of Nurse Education in the Higher Education Sector: 1994 and beyond (1994) Nursing Education in Australian Universities. AGPS.

New Zealand Health and Disability Sector Standards NS8134 NZ8134 www.acc.co.nz/ (Accessed on 29 October 2009).

Health and Disability Services Safety Act (2001) New Zealand http://www.legislation.govt.nz/act/public/2001/0093/latest/DLM119975.html (accessed on 29 October 2009).

Heath, P. National Review of Nursing Education 2002: Our Duty of Care. Department of Education, Science and Training, AGPS.

Nursing Homes Assistance Act (1974) Commonwealth http://www.austlii.edu.au/au/legis/cth/consol_act/nhaa1974271/s3a.html (accessed 21 August 2009).

Richardson, S. & Healy, J. (2004) *Who cares for our elders? What we can and can't know from existing data.* National institute of Labour Studies, Flinders University SA.

Sax Report (1978) *Nurse Education and Training: Report.* Committee of Inquiry into Nurse Education and Training to the Tertiary Education Commission, Union Offset P/L Canberra.

Senate Community Affairs Reference Committee (2002) *The patient profession – Time for action.* Report of Inquiry into Nursing. Senate Printing.

Senate Select Committee on Private Hospitals and Nursing Homes (1985). *Senate Inquiry into Nursing Homes* AGPS, Canberra.

Thompson, M. (1991) *The implementation of the ANRAC Competencies: an examination of pertinent issues* ANRAC, Canberra.

Vocational Education and Training Accreditation board (1995), *Australian Qualifications Framework (AQF)* Internet publication.

Working Group on Aged Care Worker Qualifications (2001) *Review of current role of ENs in aged care: Future directions Aged Care.* National Aged Care Forum, DOHA, Canberra.

Chapter 3

American Psychological Association. (2000). *Diagnostic and statistical manual of mental disorders – text revision* (4th ed.). Washington, DC: Author.

Antonovsky, A. (1987). *Unraveling the mystery of health.* Jossey-Bass: San Franscico.

Australian Bureau of Statistics (ABS). (2001). *Voluntary Work, Australia 2000* (Cat. No.4441.0) Canberra, ACT: Author.

Australian Bureau of Statistics (ABS). (2009). *Future population growth and ageing.* (Cat. No.4102.0) Canberra, ACT: Author.

Barrett, A.E. (1999). Social support and life satisfaction among the never married. *Research on Aging.* 21, 46-72.

Brandstädter, J., & Rothermund, K. (2002). The life-course dynamics of goal pursuit and goal adjustment: A two-process framework. *Developmental Review.* 22, 117-150.

Connidis, I. (1989). The subjective experience of aging: correlates of divergent views. *Canadian Journal of Aging.* 8, 7-18.

Crumbaugh, J. (1968). Cross-validation of Purpose-in-Life Test based on Frankl's concepts. *Journal of Individual Psychology.* 24, 74-81.

Engels, G. I., & Vermey, M. (1997). Efficacy of non-medical treatments of depression in elders: A quantitative analysis. *Journal of Clinical Geropsychology,* 3, 17-35.

Everard, K. M., Lach, H.W., Fisher, E.B., & Baum, M.C. (2000). Relationship of activity and social support to the functional health of older adults. *Journal of Gerontology: Social Science.* 55B, S208-S212.

Erikson, E. (1963). *Childhood and society.* New York: W.W. Norton.

Folkman, S., Lazarus, R.R., Pimley, S., & Novacek, J. (1987). Age differences in stress and coping processes. *Psychology and Aging,* 2, 171-184.

Garfein, A.J., & Herzog, A.R. (1995). Robust aging among the young-old, old-old, and oldest-old. *Journal of Gerontology: social Sciences.* 50B, S77-S87.

Gross, A.E., & McMullen, P.A. (1982). The help seeking process. In V.J. Delega and J. Grzelak (Eds.), Cooperation and Helping Behavior: *Theories and Research* (p. 326). New York: Academic Press.

Hertzog, C., Kramer, A.F., Wilson, R.S., & Lindenberger, U. (2009). Enrichment effects on adult cognitive development: Can the functional capacity of older adults be preserved and enhanced? *Psycholgocial Science in the Public Interest.* 9, 1-49.

Katona, C. (1993). The aetiology of depression in old age. *International Review of Psychiatry, 5,* 407-416.

Kraaij, V., Pruymboom, E., & Garnefski, N. (2002). Cognitive coping and depressive symptoms in the elderly: A longitudinal study. *Aging and mental Health,* 6, 275-281.

Keller, M.L., Leventhal, E.A., & Larson, B. (1989). Aging: The lived experience. *International Journal of Aging and Human Development.* 29, 67-82.

Lazarus, R.S., & Folkman, S. (1984). *Stress, appraisal, and coping.* New York: Springer.

Lee, G. R., & Ishu-Kintz, M. (1987). Social interaction, loneliness and emotional well-being among the elderly. *Research on Aging.* 9, 459-482.

Lemon, B.W., Bengston, V.L., & Peterson, J.A. (1972). An exploration of the activity theory of aging: Activity types and life satisfaction among in-movers to a retirement community. *Journal of Gerontology.* 27, 511-523.

Lennartsson, C., & Silverstein, J. (2001). Does engagement with life enhance survival of elderly people in Sweden? The role of social and leisure activities. *Journal of Gerontology: Social Sciences. 56B,* S335-S342.

Lindau, S.T., Schumm, L.P., Laumann, E.O., Levinson, W., O'Muircheartaigh, C.A., & Waite, L.J. (2007). A study of sexuality and health among older adults in the United States. *New England Journal of Medicine.* 357, 762-774.

Litwin, H. (2001). Social network type and morale in old age. *The Gerontologist. 41,* 516-524.

Litwin, H., & Landau, R. (2000). Social network type and social support among the old-old. *Journal of Aging Studies.* 14, 213-228.

Logan, J.R., & Spitze, G. (1994). Informal support and the use of formal services by older Americans. *Journal of Gerontology: Social Sciences. 49,* 525-534.

McCabe, M. P., Davison, T., Mellor, D., George, K., Moore, K.A., & Ski, C. (2006).Depression among older people with cognitive impairment: Prevalence and detection. *International Journal of Geriatric Psychiatry. 21,* 633-644.

Maslow, A.H. (1954). Motivation and personality. New York: Harper & Row.

Menec, V.H. (2003). The relation between everyday activities and successful aging: A 6-year longitudinal study. *Journal of Gerontology. 58B,* S74-S82.

Mence, V.H., & Chipperfield, J.G. (1997). Remaining active in later life: The role of loss of control in older adults' leisure activity participation, health, and life satisfaction. *Journal of Aging and Health. 9,* 105-125.

Mezirow, J. (1994). Understanding transformation theory. *Adult Education Quarterly, 44,* 222-232.

Moore, K.A. (2003). Development and applications of the Deakin Coping Scale. *Australian Journal of Advanced Nursing, 21* (2), 13-30.

Morrow-Howell, N., Hinterlong, J., Rozario, P.A., & Tang, F. (2003). Effects of volunteering on the wellbeing of older adults. *Journal of Gerontology. 58B,* S137-S145.

Musick, M.A., Herzog, A.R., & House, J.S. (1999). Volunteering and mortality among older adults: Findings from a national sample. *Journal of Gerontology: Social Sciences.* 54B, S173-S180.

Oman, D., Thoresen, C., & McMahon, K. (1999). Volunteerism and mortality among older adults: findings from a national sample. Journal of Health Psychology. 4, 201-316.

Peterson, C. (1999). The ticking of the social clock: Adults' beliefs about the timing of transition events. International Journal of Aging and Human Development. 142, 189-202.

Rotter, J.B. (1966). Generalised expectancies for internal versus external control of reinforcement. Psychological Monographs. 80, whole 609.

Scarmeas, N., Levy, G., Tang, M.X., Manly, J., & Stern, Y. (2001). Influence of activity on the incidence of Alzheimer's disease. Neurology. 57, 2236-2242.

Steverink, N., Westerhof, G.J., Bode, B., & Dittmann-Kohli, F. (2001). The personal experience of aging, individual resources, and subjective well-being. Journal of Gerontology: social Sciences. 56B, S364-S373.

Van Tilburg, T. (1995). Living arrangements and social arrangements of older adults. Amsterdam: Free University Press.

Van Baarsen, B. (2002). Theories on coping with loss: The impact of social support and self-esteem on adjustment to emotional and social loneliness following a partner's death in later life. Journal of Gerontology: Social Sciences. 57B, S33-S42.

Van Willigen, M. (2000). Differential benefits of volunteering across the life course. *Journal of Gerontology: Social Sciences. 55B,* 308-318.

Wenger, G.C. (1996). Social networks and gerontology. *Reviews in Clinical Gerontology. 6,* 285-293.

World Health Organisation (1947). The constitution of the World Health Organization. *WHO Chronicle, 1,* 29.

Chapter 4

* Adams, P.A., Koch, R.W. 2010 *Pharmacology: Connections to nursing practice.* New Jersey: Pearson.

Andrews-Hanna, J.R., Snyder, A.Z., et al. 2007 *Disruption of large-scale brain systems in advanced aging.* Neuron 56(5):924-935.

Austad, S.N. 2001 *Concepts and theories of aging.* in Masoro, E.J., Austad, S. *Handbook of the biology of aging.* 5th ed. UK: Academic Press.

Burton, D.G.A. 2009 *Cellular senescence, ageing and disease.* Age 31:1-9.

Chokroverty, S. 1999 *Sleep and the autonomic nervous system.* in Appenzeller, O., Vinken, P.J., G.W. Bruyn *Handbook of clinical neurology, The Autonomic nervous system Volume 74:Part 1* Oxford: Elsevier.

Connolly, M.J., Corwley, J.J., Charan, N.B., Nielson, C.P., Vestal, R.E. 1995 *Impaired bronchodilator re-*

sponse to albusterol in healthy elderly men and women. Chest 108:401-406.

Crimmins, E., Vasunilashorn, S., Kim, J.K., Alley, D. 2008 *Biomarkers related to aging in human populations.* Adv. Clin. Chem. 46:161-216.

Duffy, P.H., Feuers, R., Nakamura, K.D., Leakey, J., Hart, R.W. 1990 *Effect of chronic caloric restriction on the synchronization of various physiological measures in old female Fischer 344 rats.* Chronobiol. Int. 7(2):113-124.

Everitt, A.V., Seedsman, N.J., Jones, F. 1980 *The effects of hypophysectomy and continuous food restriction on collagen ageing, proteinuria, incidence of pathology and longevity in the make rat.* Mech. Ageing and Dev. 12:161-172.

Everitt, A.V. 1973 *The hypothalamic-pituitary control of ageing and age-related pathology.* Exp. Gerontol. 8:265-277.

Ferrara C.M., Goldberg A.P., Ortmeyer H.K., Ryan A.S. 2006 *Effects of aerobic and resistive exercise training on glucose disposal and skeletal muscle metabolism in older men.* J.Gerontology 61(5):480-7.

Ferruci, L. 2008 *The Baltimore longitudinal study of aging (BLSA):A 50-year-long journey and plans for the future.* J. Gerontology 63A(12):1416-1419.

Feuers R.J., Leakey J.E., Duffy P.H., Hart R.W., Scheving L.E. 1990 *Effect of chronic caloric restriction on hepatic enzymes of intermediary metabolism in aged B6C3F1 female mice.* Progress in Clin. and Biol. Res. 341B:177-85.

Freeman, S.H., Kandel, R., Cruz, L. et al. 2008 *Preservation of neuronal number despite age-related cortical brain atrophy in elderly subjects without Alzheimer disease.* J. Neuropath. and Exp. Neurology 67(12):1205-1212.

Goodpaster, B.H. Park, S.W., Harris, T.B. et al. for the Health ABC Study 2006 *The loss of skeletal muscle strength, mass and quality in older adults: the health, aging and body composition study. J.* Gerontology 61A(10):1059-1064.

Hastings, S.N., Purser, J.L., Johnson K.S., Sloane R.J., et al. 2008 *A frailty index predicts some but not all adverse outcomes in older adults discharged from the emergency department.* J. Am. Ger. Soc. 56(9):1651–1657.

Halverstadt A., Phares D.A., Wilund K.R., Goldberg A.P., Hagberg J.M. 2007 *Endurance exercise training raises high-density lipoprotein cholesterol and lowers small low-density lipoprotein and very low-density lipoprotein independent of body fat phenotypes in older men and women.* Metabolism 56:444-450.

Hayflick, L., Moorhead, P.S. 1961 *The serial cultivation of human diploid cell strains.* Exp. Cell Research 25:585-621.

Hofman, M.A., Swaab, D.F. 2006 *Living by the clock: The circadian pacemaker in older people.* Ageing Research Reviews 5:33–51.

Holiday, R. 1995 *Understanding ageing.* Cambridge: Cambridge Univ. Press.

Jenkins, G. 2002 *Molecular mechanisms of skin ageing.* Mech. Ageing and Dev. 123 (7):801-810.

Joosten, S.A., van Ham, V., Nolan, C.E., Borrias, M.C., Jardin, A.G., Shiels, P.G., et al. 2003 *Telomere shortening and cellular senescence in a model of chronic allograft rejection.* Am. J. Pathol. 162:1305-1312.

Joseph L.J.O., Blumenthal J., Katzel L.I., Goldberg A.P. 2005 *Exercise training and cardiovascular health with aging.* Clin. Geriatrics 13(4):40-46.

Kirkwood, T.B.L. 1977 *Evolution of aging.* Nature 270:301-304.

Kulminski, A.M. 2007 *Accelerated accumulation of health deficits as a characteristic of aging.* Exp. Gerontology, 42(10):963-70).

Kulminski, A.M., Ukrainsteva, S.V., Culminskaya, I.V., Arbeev, K.G., Land, K.C., Akushevich, L., Yashin, A.I. 2008 *Cumulative deficits and physiological indices as predictors of mortality and long life.* J. Gerontology 63A (10):1053-1059.

Lakowski, B., Hekimi, S. 1996 Determination of life-span in Caenorhabditis elegans by four clock genes. Science 272 (5264):1010-1013.

* Linton, D.L., Lach, H.W. 2007 *Matteson and McConnell's Gerontological nursing concepts and practice.* 3rd ed. Philadelphia: Saunders.

Lu, S., Y. Dai, Y. 2008 *Normal body temperature and the effects of age, sex, ambient temperature and body mass index on normal oral temperature: A prospective, comparative study.* Intl. J. Nursing Studies 46(5):661-668.

MacGibbon, M.F., Walls, R.S., Everitt, A.V. 2000 *An age-related decline in melatonin secretion is not altered by food restriction.* J. Gerontology 56A (1):B21-26.

MacGibbon, M.F. 1996 *Ageing as upregulation failure.* Medical Hypotheses 46 (6):523-528

Manda, K., Bhatia, A.L. 2004 *Melatonin-induced reduction in agerelated accumulation of oxidative damage in mice.* Biogerontology 4: 133–139, 2003.

* Masoro, E.J., Austad, S. 2006 Handbook of the biology of aging. 6th ed. UK: Academic Press.

Medawar, P.B. 1952 *An unsolved problem of biology.* London: H.K. Lewis.

Meydani, M. 1999 *Dietary antioxidants modulation of aging and immune-endothelial cell interaction.* Mech. Ageing and Dev. 111:123–132.

* Miller R.A. 1996 *The aging immune system: primer and prospectus.* Science (273) 5271.

Nakamura, E., Miyao, K. 2007 *A method for identifying biomarkers of aging and constructing and index of biological age in humans.* J. Gerontology 62A (10):1096-1105.

* Nicholl, C., Wilson, K.J., Webster, S. 2008 *Lecture notes: Elderly care medicine.* 7th ed. UK: Blackwell.

* Pikna, J.K. 2009 *Concepts of altered health in adults.* In Porth, C.M., Matfin, G. 2009 *Concepts*

of altered health states. 8th ed. Philadelphia: Lippincott, Williams and Wilkins.

* Ratnaike, R.N. (Ed.) 2002 *Practical guide to geriatric medicine.* Sydney: McGraw-Hill

Sund-Levander, M., Forsberg, C., Wahren, L.K. 2002 *Normal oral, rectal, tympanic and axillary body temperature in adult men and women: a systematic literature review.* Scand. J. of Caring Sci.16(2):122 - 128.

Tavernarakis, N. 1, Driscoll, M. 2002 *Caloric restriction and lifespan: a role for protein turnover? Mechanisms of Ageing and Development* 123:215–229.

Ungvari, Z., Parrado-Fernandez, Csiszar, Anna, De Cabo, Raphael 2008 *Mechanisms underlying caloric restriction and lifespan regulation (Review)* Circulation Res. 102:519.

Weindruch, R. 1996 *The retardation of aging by caloric restriction: studies in rodents and primates.* Toxic. Pathology 24(6):742-745.

Willcox, B.J., Willcox, D.C., Ferrucci, L. 2008 *Secrets of healthy aging and longevity from exceptional survivors around the globe: Lessons from octogenarians to supercentenarians.* J. Gerontology 63A (11):1181-1185.

Williams. G.C. 1957 *Pleiotropy, natural selection, and the evolution of senescence.* Evolution 11:398-411.

Wilson, D.M. III, Bohr, V.A., McKinnon, P.J. 2008 *DNA damage, DNA repair, ageing and age-*

elated disease. Mech. Ageing and Dev. 129 (7-8):349-352.

Chapter 5

Fergusson D, Hong B, Harwood J, et al. (2001). *Living Standards of Older New Zealanders: A summary.* Wellington: Ministry of Social Policy.

Fonda, S., Clipp, E., & Maddox, G. (2000). Patterns of functioning among residents of affordable assisted living housing facility. *Gerontologist,* 42; 178-187.

Fries, B., & Fahey, C. (2003). Introduction: Lessons learned from eight case studies. Implementing the resident assessment instrument: Case studies of policymaking for long-term care in eight countries. http://www.milbank.org/reports/interRAI/030222interRAI.html.

Hirdes, J.P., G. Ljunggren, et al. (2008). Reliability of the interRAI suite of assessment instruments: A 12-country study of an integrated health information system. *BMC Health Serv Res, 8* (1), 277.

Martin G., & Martin, I. (2003). *Assessment of community dwelling older people in New Zealand: A review of the tools.*

Ministry of Health. (1998). *Blueprint for Mental Health Services in New Zealand: How things need to be.* Author. Wellington, NZ.

Ministry of Health. (2001a). *The Primary Health Care Strategy.* Author. Wellington, NZ.

Ministry of Health. (2001b). *He Korowai Oranga – M ori Health Strategy Discussion Document.* Author. Wellington, NZ.

Ministry of Health. (2001c). *The New Zealand Palliative Care Strategy.* Author. Wellington, NZ.

Ministry of Health. (2002). *Pacific Health and Disability Action Plan.* Author. Wellington, NZ.

Ministry of Health. (2006). *Health of Older People Strategy.* Author. Wellington, NZ.

New Zealand Guidelines Group. (2003). *Assessment processes for older people.* Wellington. NZ, www.nzgg.or.nz.

Thomas, D. (2001). The critical link between health-related quality of life and aged-related changes in physical activity and nutrition. *Journal Gerontol A Biol Med Sci,* 56(10), 599-602.

Weidenbohm, K., Parsons, M., Dixon, R., Keeling, S., Brandt, T., & Kilpatrick, J. (2007). *Report 2: The interRai evaluation.*

Exploring differences of the MDS-HC trial implementation in five District Health Boards of New Zealand. Auckland UniServices Ltd, NZ.

World Health Organisation. (2007). Ten facts on aging. Retrieved March 2, 2008 from www.who.int /features/factfiles/ageing/en/index.html.

Chapter 6

Aged and Community Services Australia (2007) *The National Report.* Issue 168. Aged and Community Services Australia, 22 November.

Ballard, C., Waite, J. (2006). The effectiveness of atypical anti-psychotics for the treatment of aggression and psychosis in Alzheimer's disease. *Cochrane Database Systematic Review.* 1:1-108.

Bandura A. *Self-efficacy in changing societies.* 1995 Cambridge: Cambridge University Press.

Bowers, BL (1987) Intergenerational care-giving: Adult caregivers and their ageing parents. *Advances in Nursing Science,* 9(2):20-31.

Brooker, D. (2005) Dementia Care Mapping: a review of the research literature. *Gerontologist,* 45: 11-18.

Burke, C., Chenoweth, L and Stein-Parbury, J. (2009) The Person-Centred Environment and Care Tool. *PhD thesis.* University of Technology Sydney: Sydney, Australia.

Burns, N and Grove, SK. (2007) *Understanding Nursing Research.* 4th ed. Philadelphia: Elsevier.

Care of Older Australian Working Group (COOAWG) (2004) *National action plan for the improving the care of older people across the acute-aged care continuum.* Australian Health Ministers Advisory Council (AHMAC): Canberra, Australia. www.health.vic.gov.au/acute-ag edcare.

Chang, A. (2005) Outcomes for evidence-based nursing practice. In M Courtney (ed.) *Evidence for nursing practice.* Sydney, Australia: Elsevier. p.121.

Chenoweth, L., King, M., Jeon, Y-H., Brodaty, H., Stein-Parbury, J., Haas, M and Luscombe, G. (1999) Caring for Aged Dementia Care residents Study

(CADRES) of person-centred care, dementia care mapping and usual care in dementia: a cluster-randomised trial. *Lancet Neurology,* 8:317-25.

Chenoweth, L., Jeon, Y-H., Merlyn, T. and Brodaty, H. (2009) Factors that attract and retain nurses in aged and dementia care: A systematic literature review. *Journal of Clinical Nursing.* (in press, accepted for publication March 12, 2009).

Cochrane, AL. (1979) 1931-1971; a critical review with particular reference to the medical profession. *Medicine in the year 2000.* London: Office of Health Economics pp.1-11.

Cohen-Mansfield, J., Libin, A. and Marx, M. (2007) Nonpharmacological treatment of agitation; a controlled trial of systematic individualised intervention. J Gerontol A Bio Sci Med Sci, 62:908-16.

Courtney, M., O'Reilly, MT., Edwards, H. et al. (2007) Development of a systematic approach to developing quality within Australian residential aged care facilities. The Clinical Care Indicators (CCI) Tool. *Australian Health Review,* 31(4):582-91.

Courtney, M., C., Rickard, Vickerstaff, J. and Court, A. (2005) Evisdence-based nursing practice. In M Courtney (ed.) Evidence for nursing practice. Sydney, Australia: Elsevier. p.5-10.

Day, J., Higgins, I. and Koch, T. (2009) Delirium and older people in acute care. In R. Nay and S. Garratt (eds.) *Older people. Issues and innovations* (3rd edition). Chatswood, Australia, Churchill Livingstone, pp.244-260.

Dempsey, J. (2004) Falls prevention revisited; a call for a new approach. *Journal of Clinical Nursing,* 13: 479-85.

Donabedian, A. (1980) *The definition of quality and approaches to its assessment.* Ann Arbor, Mass. Health Administrative Press, pp.82-3.

Donabedian, A. 1988 The quality of care. How ca it be assessed? *Journal of the American Medical Association.* 260(12):1743-8.

Duffield, C., Roche, M., O'Brien-Pallas, L., Diers, D., Aisbett, C., King, M., et al. (2007). *Glueing it Together: Nurses, Their Work Environment and Patient Safety.* Sydney, Australia: NSW Department of Health.

Duncan. D., Beck, S. and Hood, J. (2006) Using dietetic assistants to improve the outcome of hip fracture: a randomised controlled trial of nutritional support in an acute trauma ward. *Age and Ageing,* 35: 148-53.

Eckwell, A., Swiberg, B., Hallberg, IR. (2004) Dimensions of informal care and quality of life among elderly family caregivers. *Scandinavian Journal of Caring Science,* 18:239-48.

Fossey, J., Ballard, C., Juszczak, E. Et al. (2006) Effect of enhanced psychosocial care on anti-psychotic use in nursing home residents with severe dementia: a cluster-randomised trial. *BMJ,* 332: 756-60.

Francke, AL, Smit, MC., de Veer, AJE. and Mistiaen, P. (2008) Factors influencing the implementation of clinical guidelines for health care professionals: A systematic review. *BMC Medical Informatics and Decision-Making,* 8: 38-48.

Gallagher, R., Donoghue, J., Chenoweth, L., Stein-Parbury, J. 2008 Self-management in older patients with chronic illness. International Journal of Nursing Practice. Vol.14(5):pp: 373-382.

Hickman, L, Phillip Newton, P and Halcombe, EJ et al. 2007 Best practice interventions to improve the management of older people in acute care settings. A literature review. Journal of Advanced Nursing, 60 (2):113-26.

Holman, H.R. & Lorig, K. (1992) Perceived self-efficacy in self-management of chronic disease, in R.E. Schwarzer (ed.), Self-efficacy: Thought control of action, vol.xiv, DC, US: Hemisphere Publishing Corp, pp.305-323.

Hsaio, JK., Jeste, DV, Katz, IR., Olin, JT, Pollock, BG., Rabins, PV., Rosenheck, RA., Small, GW., Lebowitz, B and Lieberman, JA. (2001) National Institute of Mental Health Clinical Antipsychotic Trails of Intervention Effectiveness (CATIE): Alzheimer disease trail methodology. Am. J. Geriatr Psychiatry. 9(4):346-56.

Ibe, T., Ishizaki, T., Oku, H., Ota, K., Takabatake, Y., Iseda, A., Ishikawa Y. and Ueda, A. (2008) Predictors of pressure ulcer and physical restraint prevalence in Japanese acute care units. *Japan Journal of Nursing Science,* 5(2):91-98.

Ibrahim, J., Koch, S., Holland, H. and Howie, L. (2009) Quality and safety while enhancing rights and respecting risks. In R Nay and S Garratt (eds.) *Older people. Issues and innovations.* (3rd edition) Churchill Livingstone: Sydney, Australia. pp.129-126.

Inouye, S., Leo-Summers, I., Zhang, Y. et al., (2005) A chartbased method for identification of delirium. Validation compared with interviewer ratings using the confusion assessment method. *Journal of American Geriatrics Society,* 48(12):312-8.

Institute of Medicine Committee to Advise the Public Health Service on Practice Guidelines (1990) *Clinical Practice Guidelines: Directions for a New Agency.* Washington, DC: National Academy Press.

Joanna Briggs Institute (2008) Management of constipation in older adults. *JBI Best Practice.* 12(7):1-4.

Kitson, AL., Harvey, G. and McCormack, B. (1998) Enabling the implementation of evidence-based practice: a conceptual framework. *Quality in Health Care.* 7: 149-158.

Kitson, AL., Rycroft-Malone, J., Harvey, G. et al. (2008) Evaluating the successful implementation of evidence into practice using the PARiHS framework: theoretical and practical challenges. *Implementation Science,* 3:1 published online 7 January 7. www.pubmedcentral.nih.gov/articlerender.fcgi?artid=2235887 [accessed 7 Aug 2009].

Lancet (1995) Evidence-based medicine, in its place [Editorial] *Lancet,* 346, p.785.

McCormack, J. (2008) Health care in a longevity regime. In R. Nay and S. Garrett (eds.) *Older people.*

Issues and innovations (3rd edition). Chatswood, Australia, Churchill Livingstone, pp.30-33.

McGaughan, D., Thompson, C., Callum, N., Sheldon, T and Thompson, DR. (2002) Acute care nurses' perceptions of barriers to using research information in clinical decision-making. *Journal of Advanced Nursing.* 39: 46-60.

Moorhead, S. Johnson, M., Maas, M (eds.) (2004) *Nursing Outcomes Classification* (NOC.). (3RD edition). Mosby: St Louis, USA.

Mott, B., Nolan, J., Zarb, N, et al. (2004) Clinical nurses' knowledge of evidence-based practice. Constructing a framework to evaluate a multi-faceted intervention for implementing EBP. *Contemporary Nurse,* 19:96-104.

National Health and Medical Research Council [NHMRC] (2000) How to use the evidence. Assessment and application of scientific evidence. *Handbook series on preparing clinical practice guidelines.* Commonwealth of Australia: Canberra.

National Institute for Health and Clinical Excellence (NICE) (2006) *The NICE Guidelines Manual.* London: National Institute for Health and Clinical Excellence. Available at http://www.nice.org.uk (accessed in April 2006).

Newman, M. and Roberts, T. (2002) Critical appraisal 1: is the quality of the study good enough for you to use the findings? In JV Craig and RL Smyth (eds.) *The evidence-based practice manual for nurses.* London: Churchill Livingstone. pp.109-10.

Newman, M., Thompson, C. and Roberts, AP. (2006) Helping practitioners understand the contribution of research. *Evidence-Based Nursing.* 9:4-7.

Nolan, MR., Lundh, U., Grant, G. et al., (2003) (eds.) Partnerships in family care; Understanding the care-giving career. Open University Press: Maidenhead.

Osbourne, S. & Webster, J. 2005 Development and use of evidence-based guidelines. In M Courtney (ed) *Evidence for Nursing Practice.* Marrickville, Australia: Elsevier, pp.185-9.

Parker, SG. Fadayevantan, R. and Lee, S. (2006) Acute hospital care for older people. *Age and Ageing,* 35: 551-2.

Pearson, M. and Craig, JV. (2002) Evidence-based practice in nursing. In JV Craig and RL Smyth (eds.) *The evidence-based practice manual for nurses.* London: Churchill Livingstone.

Resnick. B., Zimmerman, S., Orwig, D. et AL. (2001) Model testing for reliability and validity of the Outcome Expectations for Exercise Scale. *Nursing Research.* 50(5):293-9.

Richardson, B. and Bartlett, H. (2009) The impact of ageing-in-place policies on structural change in residential aged care. *Australasian Journal on Ageing,* 28(1):28-31.

Royal College of Nursing Australia (RCNA) (1997) Evidence-based nursing: an examination of nursing within the international evidence-based health care practice movement. Discussion Paper No.1. *Nursing Review.* pp.1-4.

Rycroft-Malone, J., Harvey, G., Seers, Kitson, A., McCormack, B. and Tichen, A. (2004) An exploration of the factors that influence the implementation of evidence into practice. *Journal of Clinical Nursing.* 13: 913-924.

Sackett, DL. and Rosenberg, WMC. (1995) On the need for evidence-based medicine. *Health Economics.* 4:249-254.

Schneider, LS., Tariot, PN., Lyketsos, CG., Dagerman, KS., Davis, KL., Davis, S.

Silagy, C. (2001) Evidence-based health care 10 years on: is the National Institute of Clinical Studies the answer? (editorial) *Medical Journal of Australia,* 175: 124-5.

Thomas, EJ. and Brennan, TA. (2000) Incidence and types of preventable adverse events in elderly patients: population review of medical records. *British Medical Journal,* 320-: 741-4.

Trinder, L. (2000) A critical appraisal of evidence-based practice. In L Trinder and S Reynolds (eds.) *Evidence-based practice. A critical appraisal.* Oxford, UK: Blackwell Science, pg. 215.

Winbolt, M., Nay, R. and Featherstonhough, D. (2009) Taking a TEAM (Translating Evidence into Aged Care Methods) approach to practice change. In R. Nay and S. Garratt (eds.) *Older people. Issues and Innovations.* (3rd edition). Chatswood, Australia: Churchill Livingstone. pp.447-9.

Chapter 7

Allan, K. & Killick, J. (2008) Communication and relationships: an inclusive social world In: Downs, M & Bowers, B (eds) Excellence in Dementia Care, McGraw Hill, Berkshire, England, pp.212-229.

Australian Institute of Health and Welfare (AIHW). Health services series no 26. Australian Hospital Statistics 2004-05. Published May 2006. Available from URL: http://www.aihw.gov.au/publications/index.cfm/title/10305.

Australian Nursing & Midwifery Council (2008). Code of Ethics for Nurses in Australia.

Australian Nursing & Midwifery Council (2008). Code of Professional Conduct for Nurses in Australia.

Conn, V., Burks, K., Rantz, M., & Knusen, K. (2002). Evidence-Based Practice for Gerontological Nursing. Journal of Gerontological Nursing 28(2) 45-52.

Davis, S., Dorevitch, M., & Garratt, S. (2009) Person-centred comprehensive geriatric assessment. In: Nay R, Garratt, S. (eds) Older People: issues and innovation in care, Churchill Livingstone, Chatswood, Australia, pp.168-188.

De Bellis, A., Bradley, S., Wotherspoon, A., Walter, B., Guein, P., Cecchin, M. & Paterson, J. (2009) Come Into My World – How to Interact with a Person who has Dementia: An educational resource for undergraduate healthcare students on person-centred care. Flinders University, Hyde Park Press, Adelaide.

Fisher, L., & Wallhagen, M. (2008). Day-to-Day Care. The Interplay of CNAs' View of Residents & Nursing Home Environments. Journal of Gerontological Nursing, 34 (11).

Fleming, M., & Kayser-Jones, J. (2008). Assuming the Mantle of Leadership. Issues and Challenges for Directors of Nursing. Journal of Gerontological Nursing 34 (11) 18-25.

Grosch, K., Medvene, L. & Woolcott, H. (2008) Person-Centred Caregiving Instruction for Geriatric Nursing Assistant Students: Development and Evaluation. Journal of Gerontological Nursing, 34 (8) 23-31.

Hughes, Julian. (2008). Being minded in dementia: persons and human beings In: Downs, M & Bowers, B. (eds) Excellence in Dementia Care, McGraw Hill, Chatswood, Australia, p124.

Hupcey, J., Clark, M., Hutcheson, C., & Thompson, V. (2004). Expectations for Care. Older Adults' Satisfaction With and Trust in Health Care Providers. Journal of Gerontological Nursing 30 (11) 37-45.

Ibrahim, J., Koch, S., Holland, A., & Howie, L. (2009). Quality and safety while enhancing rights and respecting risk. In: Nay, R. and Garratt, S. (eds) Older People: issues and innovation in care, Churchill Livingstone, Chatswood, Australia, pp.168-188.

International Council of Nurses (2006). The ICN Code of Ethics for Nurses. www.icn.ch/icncode.pdf.

Kilshaw, Lucy. (2009). Australian and New Zealand Society for Geriatric Medicine. Position Statement No.14. Guidelines for the Management of Older Persons Presenting to Emergency Departments 2008. *Australasian Journal of Ageing* Vol 28: 3. 153-157.

Kitwood, T. (1997). Person and Process in Dementia. International Journal of Geriatric Psychiatry, 8, 541-545.

Lim, W.K., Cong, C., Caplan, G, and Gray, L. (2009). Australian and New Zealand Society for Geriatric Medicine. Position Statement No.15. Discharge Planning.

McCormack, B. (2004). Person-centredness in Gerontological nursing: An overview of the literature. International Journal of Older People Nursing, 13(13a), 31-38.

McCormack, B (2003). A conceptual framework for personcentred practice with older people. International Journal of Nursing Practice, 9: 203-209.

McCormack, B., & McCance, T. (2006). Development of a framework for person-centred nursing. Journal of Advanced Nursing 56 (5) 472-479.

Moehead, A., Barraclough, F & Alavi, C (2008) A positive approach to the care of the older person: Final report, report to North Coast Area Health Service; Southern Cross University, Lismore, NSW.

Mullins, L. & Hartley, T. (2002). Residents' Autonomy: Nursing Home Personnel's Perceptions. Journal of Gerontological Nursing 28(2), 35-44.

New Zealand Ministry of Health (2002b) *Health of Older people: Health sector action to 2010 to support positive ageing.* Ministry of Health, Wellington.

New Zealand Ministry of Health (2004) *New Zealand Guideline for Specialist Health Services for Older People.* Ministry of Health. Wellington.

Nolan, L. (2006). Caring connections with older persons with dementia in an acute hospital setting – a hermeneutic interpretation of the staff nurse's experience. International Journal of Older People Nursing, 1 (4) 208-213.

Nursing Council of New Zealand (2008). Code of Conduct for Nurses.

Registered Nurses Association of Ontario. (2002) Client Centred Care. *Best Practice Guidelines Project. Shaping the Future of Nursing, Toronto.* Available from URL: www.rnao.org.

Rogers, C. (2008). Carl Rogers.info – resources for students, researchers and practitioners. Accessed 13 July 2009, from http://www.carlrogers.info/book sabout.html

Thompson, F., Girling, D., Green, S., & Wai, C. (2008). Care of people with dementia in the general hospital. In: Downs, M & Bowers, B (eds) Excellence in Dementia Care, McGraw Hill, Berkshire, England, pp.301-318.

Thompson, I., Melia, K. & Boyd K. (eds) (2000) Nursing and Nursing Ethics into the 21st Century In: Nursing Ethics, Churchill Livingstone, London, England, 4th edn. p.328.

Walent, R., & Kayser-Jones, J. (2008) Having a Voice and Being Heard. Journal of Gerontological Nursing 34 (11), 34-42.

Chapter 8

Aboderin, I., Kalache, A., Ben-Shlomo, Y., Lynch, J.W., Yajnik, C.S., Kuh, D., Yach, D. (2002) *Life Course Perspectives on Coronary Heart Disease, Stroke and Diabetes: Key Issues and Implications for Policy and Research.* Geneva, World Health Organization.

Acute Coronary Care Working Group guidelines for the management of acute coronary syndromes 2006 MJA; 184 (8 Suppl):S1-S32.

Australian Institute of Health and Welfare (AIHW) (2006). Australian incontinence data analysis and development. AIHW cat. No.DIS 44. Canberra.

Australian Institute of Health and Welfare (AIHW) Senes, S 2006. How we manage stroke in Australia.

Australian Institute of Health and Welfare (AIHW) AIHW Cited National Continence Management Strategy Evaluation Framework January 2009.

Australian Institute of Health and Welfare (AIHW) and the National Breast and Ovarian Cancer Centre. Breast Cancer in Australia: An Overview, 2009.

Australian Institute of Health and Welfare (AIHW) Older Australians at a glance Edition 4 – Health and functioning (November 2007).

Australian Institute of Health and Welfare (AIHW) Cancer survival and prevalence in Australia Cancers diagnosed from 1982 to 2004 Cancer Australia and the Australasian Association of Cancer registries July 2008.

Australian Institute of Health and Welfare (AIHW) Hospitalisations due to falls by older people, Australia 2005–06.

Australian Institute of Health and Welfare (AIHW) 2008. A picture of osteoporosis in Australia. Arthritis series no.6. Cat. no.PHE 99. Canberra: AIHW.

Australian Institute of Health and Welfare (AIHW) Injury Research and Statistics Series Number 50 Canberra Cat. no.INJCAT 122.

Broe, Prof T. (2009) unpublished proceedings of Growing Old Well – Inaugural National AAG AAC Workshop, Sydney 2008.

Brown, Peter. (ed) Health Care and the Aged – a Nursing perspective (2 nd ed) 1994.

Brown, D and Edwards, H. (2005) Lewis's Medical Surgical Nursing, Assessment and Management of Clinical Problems. Elsevier, Aust.

Cadilhac, D., H. Dewey et al. Investing in Stroke – What are the potential cost offsets from the strokesafe program. National Stroke Research Institute – Technical Report (Unpublished) 2005.

Carmody, Susan and Forster, Sue. Aged Care Nursing – A guide to Practice Ausmed Publications 2003.

Close, Dr Jacqui – presentation for Australian Association of Gerontology (AAG) 2006 'Fall and Ageing in Place'.

Cotter, P. Anderson, I and Smith, L. Indigenous Australians: Ageing without Longevity (2007) cited in

Borowski, A. Encel, S and Ozanne, E Longevity and Social Change in Australia UNSW Press.

Dunning, T. (2005) Nursing Care of Older People with Diabetes, Wiley-Blackwell.

Francis, (Deborah C. 2009) MSN APRN BC Geriatric Clinical Nurse Specialist Kaiser Permanente Medical Center South Sacramento, CA http://consultgerirn.org/about.

Gillespie LD, Robertson MC, Gillespie WJ, Lamb SE, Gates S, Cumming RG, Rowe BH. Interventions for preventing falls in older people living in the community. *Cochrane Database of Systematic Reviews* 2009, Issue 2. Art. No.: CD007146. DOI: 10.1002/14651858.CD007146.pub2.

Higgins, I., Madjar, I., and Walton, J.A. (2004). Chronic pain in elderly nursing home residents: the need for nursing leadership. Journal of nursing management, 12, 167-173.

Hogan, A. O'Loughlin, K. Miller, P and Kendig, H. (2009) The Health Impact of a Hearing Disability on Older People in Australia Journal of Aging and Health Vol 21 no 8.

JBI Model of Evidence-Based Healthcare. Strategies to reduce medication errors with reference to older adults.

JBI Management of constipation in older adults *Best Practice* 12(7) 2008 | Volume 12 Issue 7 2008 ISSN: 1329-1874.

Jones V., MD, Berkwits, Michael, MD, Kaplan, Justin L., MD, and Porter, Robert, MD The Merck Manual of

Health & Aging, Merck Research Labs, Division of Merck and Co., Inc. Whitehouse Station, NJ 2004.

Lord, S. (2005) Vision Balance and Falls in the Elderly. Geriatric Times Volume 6 issue 6.

Leipzig RM, Cumming RG, Tinetti ME Drugs and falls in older people: A systematic review and meta-analysis: I Psychotropic drugs J Am Geriatr Soc 1999 47: 30-39.

Lewis SJ, Heaton KW (1997). 'Stool form scale as a useful guide to intestinal transit time'. Scand. J. Gastroenterol. 32 (9):920–4.

(Liu CJ, Latham NK. Progressive resistance strength training for improving physical function in older adults. Cochrane Database of Systematic Reviews 2009, Issue 3. Art. No.: CD002759. DOI: 10.1002/14651858.CD002759.pub2).

Lord, Sherrington, Menz, Close Falls in older people: risk factors and strategies for prevention Cambridge University Press. (2001).

McNeil, MEA The First Year – Rheumatoid Arthritis An essential guide for the Newly Diagnosed, Marlow and Company, New York 2005.

Mitchell P, Taylor HR, Keeffe JE, Vu H, Wang JJ, Rochtchina E, Pezzullo LM, 'Vision Loss in Australia' Medical Journal of Australia 2005v12 (11) pp.565-568.

Milton, James C. Hill-Smith, Ian and Jackson, Stephen H D. BMJ 2008;336;606-609 doi:10.1136/bmj.39503.424653.80.

Ministry of Health, New Zealand. (2002). Health of Older People Strategy.

Nay Rhonda and Garratt, Sally Older people Issues and Innovations, 3rd Edition 2009 Elsevier, Australia.

NSW Ministerial Advisory committee on ageing (2003). Hear all about it. Proceedings of Public consultation.

O'Neill, P Caring for the Older Adult – A Health Promotion Perspective (2002) Saunders, USA.

RACGP and The National Stroke Foundation, (2008) Clinical Guidelines for Stroke and TIA Management: A guide for general practice.

RACGP, National Heart Foundation and The Cardiac Society of Australia and New Zealand. Guidelines for the Management of Acute Coronary Syndromes Medical Journal of Australia Volume 184 Number 8.

Rawlings-Anderson, K and Johnson, K. (2003) Myocardial infarction and older people. Nursing older People. Sep;15(6):29-34.

Redfern, S and Ross, F. (4th Ed 2006) Nursing Older People. Elsevier (Churchill Livingstone) UK.

Report prepared by the Australian Patient Safety Foundation for the National Health Priorities and Quality Branch of the Department of Health and Aged Care of the Commonwealth Government of Australia August 2001 http://www.apsf.net.au/dbfiles/Iatrogenic_Injury.pdf.

Runciman B, Merry A, and Walton M. Safety and ethics in health care: a guide to getting it right. Aldershot: Ashgate, 2007.

Sambrook, Philip N. Seeman, Ego, Phillips, Stephen R and Ebeling, Peter R. Preventing osteoporosis:

outcomes of the Australian Fracture Prevention Summit (2002) Medical Journal of Australia.

Scott, Dr Sophie. Live a Longer life The Scientific Secrets for health and wellbeing at any age. (2007) ABC books.

Simons LA, Simons J, Friedlander Y, McCallum J. Does a diagnosis of the metabolic syndrome provide additional prediction of cardiovascular disease and total mortality in the elderly? The Dubbo Study Med J Aust 2007;186:400-403.

Simons LA, Simons J, Friedlander Y, McCallum J. Usefulness of fasting plasma glucose to predict mortality or coronary heart disease in persons ≥60 years of age without diabetes mellitus or in those with undiagnosed diabetes mellitus (from the Dubbo Study) Am J Cardiol 2008;102:831-834.

Singh, N. Clements, K and Fiatorone, M (1997)A randomized Control Trial of Progressive Resistance Training in Depressed Elders Journal of Gerontology 52A (1) M27 – M35.

Smith, J. Mitchell, P. Wang, Jie Jin. Leeder, S. (2005) Health policy for hearing impairment in older Australians: what should it include? Australia and New Zetland Health Policy.

Thrift AG, Dewey HM, Macdonell RAL, McNeil JJ, Donnan GA 2000. Stroke incidence on the East Coast of Australia: the North East Melbourne Stroke Incidence Study (NEMESIS). Stroke 31 (9):2087-2092.

Wallis, M. (2003) Preventing faecal incontinence through prevention and management of constipation in adults aged 40-65 years: Developing and evaluating guidelines for health professionals and resources for their clients. Final report prepared for the Australian Government Department of Health and Ageing.

Wilson, LA (2005) Understanding Bowel Problems in Older People Nov; 17(8):25-9.

Webster's New World Medical Dictionary., 3rd edition (May, 2008) Wiley Publishing, Inc.; ISBN-10: 0470189282; ISBN-13: 978-0470189283.

Chapter 9

Ackland, M & Catford, J (2004) *Measuring Population Health Status in Australia.* In Helen Keller and Berni Murphy Understanding Health: A Determinants Approach. Oxford University Press Australia.

American Psychiatric Association (2005) Diagnostic and Statistical Manual of Mental Disorders 4th Ed. Washington: APA.

Ames, D., & Ritchie, C. (2007). Psychiatric Disorders Affecting the Elderly in Australia. In G. Meadows, B. Sing, & M. Grigg, *Mental Health in Australia: Collaborative Community Practice* (2nd Edition ed., pp.450-459). Melbourne: Oxford University Press.

Anderson, D.N. (2001) Treating depression in old age: the reasons to be positive. *Age and Ageing,* 30 13-17.

Andrew, P., & Page, A.C. (2005). Outcome measurements, outcome management and monitoring.

Australian and New Zealand Journal of Psychiatry, 649.

Audin, K., Margison, F., Clark, J., & Barkham, M. (2001). Value of HoNOS in assessing patient change in NHS psychotherapy and psychological treatment services. *British Journal of Psychiatry, 178,* 561-566.

Australian Government. (2008). *Health across the life stages.* Retrieved January 21, 2009, from Australian's national agency for health and welfare statistics and information: www.aihw.gov.au.

Australian Government (2005). The Cornell Scale for Depression in Dementia. Administration & Scoring Guidelines. Department of Health and Ageing. Downloaded 25 October, 2009 from http://www.he alth.gov.au.

Baldwin, R.C., Chiu, E., Katona, C., Graham, N. (2002). *Guidelines on Depression in Older People.* London: Martin Dunitz.

Burns, A., Beevor, A., Lelliott, P., Wing, J., Blakey, A., Orrell, M., et al. (1999). Health of a Nation Outcome Scales for Elderly People (HoNOS 65+). *The British Journal of Psychiatry,* 424-427.

Butcher, H.K & McGonigal-Kennedy, M. (2005). Depression and dispiritedness in late life: A 'grey drizzle of horror' isn't inevitable. Australian Journal of Nursing, 105 (12), 52-61.

Commonwealth Department of Health and Aged Care. (2000). *National Action Plan for Promotion, Prevention and Early Intervention for Mental Health.*

Canberra: Commonwealth Department of Health and Aged Care.

Draper, B., Melding, P. and Brodaty, H. (2007). Psychogeriatric service delivery. An international perspective. Oxford: Oxford University Press.

Fortinash. K (2004). *The Schizophrenias* Chapter 11 In Katherine Fortinash and Patricaia Holoday Worret's Psychiatric Mental Health Nursing. (3rd ed.). Morsby Missouri.

Folstein MF, Folstein SE, McHugh PR. (1975) Mini-mental state: a practical method for grading the cognitive state of patients for the clinician. *Journal of Psychiatric Research* 12: 189-198.

Hansson, L. (2006). Determinents of quality of life in people with severe mental illness. *Acta Psychiatr Scand,* 113, 46-50.

Hassett, A., Ames, D., Chiu, E. (2005) *Psychosis in the Elderly,* London: Taylor and Francis.

Hazelton, M. (2001). Assessing mental health. Chapter 6. In Susan Koch and Sally Garratt Assessing Older People: a practical guide for health professionals. Mac Lennan & Petty Pty Limited. Australia.

Heffern, W.A. (2000) Psychological and electroconvulsive treatment of anxiety and depression in the elderly. *Journal of Psychiatric and Mental Health Nursing,* 7, 199-204.

Hibberd, J., & Hong, C.S. (2007). The importance of outcome measures in elderly care. *International Journal of Therapy and Rehabilitation,* 14 (5), 248.

Howart, P., Duncan, B., & Horner, B. (2004). Promoting the health of older Australians: program options, priorities and research. *Australian Health Review,* 49-55.

Inouye, S.K., van Dyck, C.H., Alessie, C.A., Balkin, S.M, Horwitz, R.I (1990) Clarifying confusion: the Confusion assessment Method. *Annals of Internal Medicine* 113:941-948.

Jacob, A., Prasad, S., Boggild, M. And Chandratre, S. (2004). Charles-Bonet Syndrome - elderly people and visual hallucinations. British Medical Journal, 328, 1552-1554.

Lebret, S., Perret-Vaille, E., Mulliez, A., Gerbaud, L. Jalenques, I. (2006) Elderly suicide attempters: characteristics and outcome. *International Journal of Geriatric Psychiatry,* 21:1052–1059.

McDonald, R., & Brown, P. (2008). Exploration of social support systems for older adults: A preliminary study. *Contemporary Nurse,* 29 (2), 184-194.

McKay, R., McDonald R. (2008). Experisive detour or a way forward? The experience of routine outcomes measures in aged care psychiatry. *The Royal Australian and New Zealand College of Psychiatry* 16 (6).

Meadows, G., & Fossey, F. (2007). A structured assessment instrument as a guide to essential skills. In G. Meadows, B. Singh, & M. Grigg, *Mental Health in Australia: Collaborative Community Practice* (pp. 296-309). Melbourne: Oxford University Press.

Mendes de Leon, C., Glass, T., & Berkman, L. (2003). Social Engagement and Disability in a Community Population of Older Adults. *Americal Journal of Epidemiology,* 157 (7), 6332-642.

Murphy, K.P. (2004). Delirium, Dementia, and Amnestic and Other Cognitive Disorders Chapter 14 In Katherine Fortinash and Patricia Holoday Worret's Psychiatric Mental Health Nursing. (3rd ed.). Morsby Missouri.

Newman, D.W., Kellett, S., & Beail, N. (2003). From research and development to practice-based evidence: clinal goverence initiative in a service for adults with mild intellectual disability and mental health needs. *Journal of Intellectual Disability Research,* 47 (1), 68-74.

NSW Department of Health (2003). Suicide prevention in older people: Training Manual. Sydney: NSW Department of Health www.health.nsw.gov.au.

Pirkis, J., Burgess, P., Kirk, P., Dodson, S., Coombes, T., & Williamson, M. (2005). A review of the psychometric properties of the Health of a Nation Outcome Scales (HoNOS) family of measures. *Health and Quality of Life Outcomes.*

Reichstadt, J., Depp, C., Palinkas, L., Folsom, D., & Jeste, D. (2007). Building Blocks of Successful Aging: A Focus Group Study of Older Adults' Perceived Contributions to Successful Aging. *American Journal of Geriatric Psychiatry,* 15 (3), 194-201.

Rowland, J.T., Basic, D., Storey, J.E., Conforti, D. (2006) The Rowland Universal Dementia Assessment

Scale (RUDAS) and the Folstein MMSE in a multicultural cohort of elderly persons *International Psychogeriatrics* 18(1), 111-120.

Sadock, B.J., Sadock, V.A. (2007). *Kaplan & Sadock's Synopsis of Psychiatry.* Philadelphia: Lippincott Williams & Wilkins.

Sharp, L.K., Lipsky, M.S. (2002). Screening for Depression across the lifespan: A review of measures for use in primary care settings. *American Family Physician* 66(6):1001-1008.

Shulman, K. (2000) Clock-drawing: is it the ideal cognitive screening test? *International Journal of Geriatric Psychiatry,* 15:548-61.

Singh, N.A., Clements, K.M., Fiatarone, M.A. (1997) A randomised controlled trial of progressive resistance training in depressed elders. *Journal of Gerontology: Medical Sciences,* 52A(1), M27-M35.

Slade, M. (2002). Routine outcome assessment in mental health services. 32, 1339-1343.

Snowdon, J. (2001) Late-life depression: what can be done? *Australian Prescriber* 24(3), 65-67.

Tansella, M., & Thornicroft, G. (2001). *Mental Health Outcome Measures* (2nd Edition ed.). London: Gaskell, The Royal College of Psychiatrists.

The New South Wales Institute of Psychiatry (2007). Older adults: Overview of the literature. Monograph 4 in A. O'Hanlon, A Patterson & J Parham (Series Eds), *Promotion, Prevention and Early Intervention for Mental Health in General Practice.* Adelaide: Australian Network for Promotion, Prevention and Early Intervention for Mental Health (Ausinet).

Turvey, C., Conwell, Y., Jones, M., Phillips, C., Simonsick, E., Pearson, J., et al. (2002). Risk Factors for Late-Life Suicide: A Prospective, Community-Based Study. *American Journal of Geriatric Psychiatry,* 10, 398-406.

Uchino, B. (2006). Social Support and Health: A Review of Physiological Processes Potentially Underlying Links to Disease. *Journal of Behavioural Medicine,* 29 (4), 377-387.

Van der Wurff, F.B., Stek, M.L., Hoogendijk, W.J.G., Beekman, A.T.F. (2003). The efficacy and safety of ECT in depressed older adults: A literature review. *International Journal of Geriatric Psychiatry.* 18(10):894-904.

Yesavage, J. (1993) Differential Diagnosis between Depression and Dementia, *American Journal of Medicine* 94: 5A-235.

Chapter 10

Australian Government (2007). Atypical anti-psychotic agents and extrapyramidal side effects. Australian Adverse Drug Reactions Bulletin, 26, 4. Department of Health and Ageing Therapeutic Goods Administration.

Australian Government (2008). Medication management reviews. Department of Health and Ageing.

Australian Government (2007). Aripiprazole and neuroleptic malignant syndrome. Australian Adverse

Drug Reactions Bulletin, 26, 2. Department of Health and Ageing Therapeutic Goods Administration.

Australian Medicine Handbook Drug Choice Companion: Aged Care, 2006, 2nd Ed.

Barry, M.D. and Cusack, J. (2004). Pharmacokinetics in older persons. The American Journal of Geriatric Pharmacotherapy, 2, 4, 274-302.

Beardsley, R.S., Kimberlin, C.L. and Tindall, W.N. (2007). Communication skills in pharmacy practice. Baltimore: Lippincott Williams & Wilkins.

Boon, N.A., Colledge, N.R. and Walker, B.R. (2006). Davidson's principles and practice of medicine. 20th ed. Philadelphia: Elsevier.

Bressler, R. and Bahl, J.J. (2003). Principles of drug therapy for the elderly patient. Mayo Clinic Proceedings. http://www.clinicalproceedings.com/content/78/12/1564.full.pdf.

Burton ME, Shaw LM, Schentag JJ, Evans, WE. *Applied Pharmacokinetics and Pharmacodynamics: principles of therapeutic drug monitoring,* Lippincott Williams & Wilkins, 2006, 4th Ed.

Corallo, C.E. and Ernest, D. Atypical neuroleptic malignant syndrome. Critical Care and Resuscitation, 9, 338-340.

Davison, A.M., Cameron, S.J., Grunfeld, J-P., Ponticelli, C., Ritz, E., Winearls, C. And van Persele, C. (eds.) (2005). Oxford textbook of clinical nephrology. Oxford: Oxford University Press.

Ebersole, P., Hess, P., Touhy, T. And Jet, K. (2008). Gerontological nursing and healthy aging. USA: Elsevier.

George, J., Kong, D.C.M., Thoman, R. and Stewart, K. (2005). Factors associated with medication nonadherence in patients with COPD. Chest, 128, 5, 3198-3204.

Halter J.B., Ouslander JG, Tinetti ME, Studenski S, High KP, Asthana S. *Hazzard's Geriatric Medicine and Gerontology,* McGraw Hill, 2009, 6th Ed.

Hilmer, S.N. (2008). The dilemma of polypharmacy. Australian Prescriber, 31, 2-3.

Hilmer, S.N., Shenfield, G.M. and Le Couteur, D.G. (2005). Clinical implications of changes in hepatic drug metabolism in older people. Therapeutic Clinical Risk Management, 1, 2, 151-156.

Hunter Division of General Practice (2007). Audit of use of psychotropic medication in residential aged care facilities. http://www.gpaccess.com.au. Downloaded 28 October, 2009.

Isbister, G.K., Buckley, N.A. and Whyte, I.M. (2007). Serotonin toxicity: a practical approach to diagnosis and treatment. *eMJA,* 187, 6, 361-365.

Junius-Walker, U., Theile, G. and Hummers-Pradier, E. (2007). Prevalence and predictors of polypharmacy among older primary care patients in Germany, 24, 1, 14-19.

Mangoni, A.A. and Jackson, S.H.D. (2004). Age-related changes in pharmacokinetics and pharmacodynamics: basic principles and practical applications. British Journal of Clinical Pharmacology, 57, 1, 6-14.

Merle, L., Laroche, M-L., Dantoine, T. And Charmes, J-P. (2005). Predicting and preventing adverse drug reactions in the very old. Grugs and Aging, 22, 5, 375-392.

National Prescribing Service Ltd. (2007) Managing osteoarthritic pain. http://www.nps.org.au/consumers/publications/medicines_talk/mt22/managing_the_pain_of_osteoarthritis. Downloaded 28 October 2009.

Noble, R.E. (2003). Drug therapy in the elderly. Metabolism, 52, 2, 27-30.

Patient UK (2008). Prescribing for the older patient. http://www.patient.co.uk.doctor/Prescribing-for-the-Older-Patient.htm.

Pharmaceutical Society of Australia. Checklist for medication history. http://www.psa.org.au/site.php?id=3445. Downloaded 28 October, 2009.

Pharmacy Guild of Australia. Module 5 – Medication and continence. http://www.novapolicy.com/pccp/PDF/MODULES-MEDICATION_AND_CONTINENCE.pdf.

Pirmohamed, M., James, S., Meakin, C., Green, A.K., Scott, T.J. Walley, K. Farrar, B.K. Park, and A.M. Breckenridge (2004). Adverse drug reactions as cause of admission to hospital: prospective analysis of 18 820 patients. British Medical Journal, 329, 15-19.

Ratnaike, R.N. and Ratnaike, RN. (2002) Practical guide to geriatric medicine. McGraw Hill.

Read, K. And Purse, M. (2009). Extrapyramidal side effects. About.Com: bipolar disorder. http://www.bipolar.about.com/od/glossary/g/gl_extrapyramid.htm.

Roughead, E.E. (2005). Managing adverse drug reactions: time to get serious. *eMJA,* 182, 6, 264-265.

Snowdon, J., Day, S., Baker, W. Current use of psychotropic medication in nursing homes. *International Psychogeriatrics.* 2006; 18:241-250.

The Merck Manual Online Medical Library. Distribution. http://www.merck.com/mmhe/sec02/ch011/ch01d.html. Downloaded 1 November, 2009.

The Merck Manual Online Medical Library. Pharmacokinetics in the elderly. http://www.merck.com/mmpe/sec20/ch306/ch306b.html. Downloaded 1 November, 2009.

The Merck Manual Online Medical Library. Precautions with over the counter drugs. http://www.merck.com/mmke/sec02/ch018b.html. Downloaded 1 November, 2009.

The Royal Australian College of General Practitioners (2005). Medical care of older persons in residential aged care facilities. 4th ed. The Royal Australian College of General Practitioners.

Woodward, M., Elliott, R., Vernon, G, Tanner, F. And Saunders, R. (2006). Beta-blockers for treatment of heart failure in the elderly. Journal of Pharmacy Practice and Research, 36, 3, 229-233.

Wynne, H. (2005). Drug metabolism and ageing. Menopause International, 11, 51-56.

Yurnheim, K. (2003). When drug therapy gets old: pharmacokinetics and pharmacodynamics in the elderly. Experimental Gerontology, 38, 8, 843-853.

Other books available from Woodslane Press

How to Master Nursing Calculations

Pass numeracy tests and make sense of drug dosage charts

To promote safe practice, nursing schools test for basic arithmetic both at interview stage and during the 3 years of nurse training. How to Master Nursing Calculations will help you to cope with these tests, offering a step-by-step approach which will take you from base-level knowledge to competency both in drug calculations and the ability to read drug dosage charts. The book begins with a helpful diagnostic section which will help you to identify your strengths and weaknesses, before going on to cover basic numeracy. It goes on to deal with drug dosage calculations and prescription awareness questions at both basic and more advanced levels. You are therefore able to take a measured and progressive approach to your learning. It features clear illustrations showing how to read instrument scales, medical admin records and pharmaceutical labels. Combining drug dosage charts, a chapter on drug administration (including a list of abbreviations and their meanings), mock tests with answers and full explanations, How to Master Nursing Calculations will be an essential asset during your years as a trainee nurse – and beyond.

Caring for Your Elderly Parent

A guide for Australian families

Most people will be involved at some stage in helping older adults, be their parents, siblings, spouse, other relatives or friends. They may need to simply help make important decisions about their health, housing, personal and physical care, and their financial and legal affairs, or they may be giving far more extensive hands-on assistance and care. Very often we come to this role of carer or adviser with little experience or knowledge of what it means to be growing older and more frail, what kind of care they might need, what care is available and how to access it. This new book has been written expressly to help any Australian who finds themselves in this situation, or wants to prepare for that time.

Feedback

We do hope that you have found this book useful, but we know that nothing in this world is perfect and your suggestions for improving future editions would be much appreciated.

Your name: _____

Your address or email address:_____

Your contact phone (optional): _____

What you most liked about Health Care of the Older Adult:

[space left intentionally blank in the original book]

What you least liked about the book: _____

[space left intentionally blank in the original book]

Please tick below and return this form (or simply email us the salient details) if you would like to be kept informed of Woodslane's products and services:

[ ] notifications of new editions of this book

[ ] details of other nursing books published by Woodslane Press

[ ] details of other nursing and medical books distributed by Woodslane

Woodslane Pty Ltd, 7/5 Vuko Place, Warriewood NSW 2102 Tel: 02-9970-5111 Fax: 02-9970-5002

Email: info@woodslane.com.au

Back Cover Material

HEALTH CARE OF THE OLDER ADULTE

An Australian and New Zealand nursing perspective

Age, and the meaning of old age have changed dramatically over the past century. Average life expectancies in Australia and New Zealand have increased dramatically and, as a result, the number of people aged 65 years and over now makes up 12-13% of both populations. This trend will continue as the "Baby Boomers" (born 1946-1964) age.

This book sets out to describe the issues and consequences of this increasingly ageing population on the Nursing profession in both Australia and New Zealand. It is suitable as a key textbook for all students of nursing, for qualified nurses working in care of the older adult, and for carers and readers with an interest in aged care.

Chapters and features include:

- Understanding people's experience of ageing
- Policy issues in relation to aged care in Australia and New Zealand
- The psychology of ageing
- Biological ageing and functional system changes
- Health Assessment of the older adult in Aotearoa NZ
- Evidence-based nursing practice – why research is necessary

- Person-centred care and the uniqueness of the individual
- Common health problems of old age
- Mental Health and illness in old age
- Clinical Pharmacology and older adults
- Exercises and Case Studies throughout

The Editor, **Dr. Peter Brown,** has worked in various Universities in NSW over a 25-year span as a Lecturer, Senior Lecturer, and Assistant Head of School. His specialty areas and interests include mental health problems in old age, aged care, and mental health, and he has lectured in these at undergraduate and post-graduate level. He has also lectured a multidisciplinary postgraduate course at the NSW Institute of Psychiatry. He has edited two textbooks on aged care and presented numerous conference papers, both nationally and internationally.

A

B

D

E

F

G

H

I

J

K

L

M

Q

R

S

T

W

Books For ALL Kinds of Readers

At ReadHowYouWant we understand that one size does not fit all types of readers. Our innovative, patent pending technology allows us to design new formats to make reading easier and more enjoyable for you. This helps improve your speed of reading and your comprehension. Our EasyRead printed books have been optimized to improve word recognition, ease eye tracking by adjusting word and line spacing as well as minimizing hyphenation. Our EasyRead SuperLarge editions have been developed to make reading easier and more accessible for vision-impaired readers. We offer Braille and DAISY formats of our books and all popular E-Book formats.

Printed in Dunstable, United Kingdom

91342610R00228